ROBERT S. PORTER

BRADY

INTERMEDIATE
EMERGENCY CARE
SECOND EDITION

BRYAN E. BLEDSOE, D.O., EMT-P
Medical Director, Emergency Department
Baylor Medical Center—Ellis County
Waxahachie, Texas
and
Clinical Associate Professor of Emergency Medicine
University of North Texas Health Sciences Center
Fort Worth, Texas

RICHARD A. CHERRY, M.ED., NREMT-P
Director of Paramedic Training
Department of Emergency Medicine
State University of New York Health Science Center
Syracuse, New York

ROBERT S. PORTER, M.A., NREMT-P
Senior Advanced Life Support Educator
Madison County Emergency Medical Service
Canastota, New York

BRADY
PRENTICE HALL
UPPER SADDLE RIVER, NEW JERSEY 07458

ACKNOWLEDGMENT

Special thanks to the following reviewers, whose special attention to detail helped ensure the content accuracy of this manual:

Edward B. Kuvlesky, NREMT-P, Battalion Chief, Indian River County EMS, Indian River, FL; and **Craig N. Story**, NREMT-P, Polk Community College, Winter Haven, FL

PUBLISHER: *Susan Katz*
MANAGING DEVELOPMENT EDITOR: *Lois Berlowitz*
DEVELOPMENT EDITOR: *Deborah Parks*
EDITORIAL ASSISTANT: *Carol Sobel*
MARKETING MANAGER: *Judy Streger*
DIRECTOR OF MANUFACTURING & PRODUCTION: *Bruce Johnson*
MANUFACTURING BUYER: *Ilene Sanford*
MANAGING PRODUCTION EDITOR: *Patrick Walsh*
PRODUCTION EDITOR: *Julie Boddorf*
PRODUCTION SUPERVISION: *Navta Associates, Inc.*
INTERIOR DESIGN: *Barbara J. Barg*
PRINTER/BINDER: *Banta Company, Harrisonburg, Virginia*

Printed in the United States of America
10 9 8 7

ISBN 0-8359-5263-0

Prentice-Hall International (UK) Limited, *London*
Prentice-Hall of Australia Pty. Limited, *Sydney*
Prentice-Hall Canada Inc., *Toronto*
Prentice-Hall Hispanoamericana, S.A., *Mexico*
Prentice-Hall of India Private Limited, *New Delhi*
Prentice-Hall of Japan, Inc., *Tokyo*
Pearson Education Asia Pte. Ltd., *Singapore*
Editoria Prentice-Hall do Brasil, *Ltda., Rio de Janero*

NOTICE ON CARE PROCEDURES

CONTENTS

INTERMEDIATE EMERGENCY CARE

Welcome to the Self-Instructional Workbook for *Intermediate Emergency Care,* Second Edition. You can use this self-instructional workbook either as a stand-alone workbook or with instructor supervision. It addresses the National Standard Curriculum for Intermediate training and meets the content described by the DOT Objectives.

This workbook is designed to help you identify the important principles presented in *Intermediate Emergency Care* and direct you to review any material you don't truly understand. The workbook addresses each case study presented in the text and explains why certain aspects of care are offered. Self-examinations test your reading comprehension and prepare you for the tests within your training course and for state examination.

Some of the features of this self-instructional workbook include:

OBJECTIVE REVIEW

Each chapter of the workbook begins with a short review of the focus of each learning objective. Use these objectives and the associated comments to identify what is important to learn during your reading of *Intermediate Emergency Care.*

CASE STUDY REVIEW

The workbook reviews the case study beginning each chapter of the text. It identifies principles and special considerations of care. It can help you learn about the elements of field care associated with each chapter of the text.

CONTENT REVIEW

Each chapter contains between 5 and 45 questions that test your comprehension. Take each self-exam carefully and then check your answers against the key in the back of this workbook. Review any questions that you may miss.

SPECIAL PROJECTS

The workbook includes several special projects that challenge your knowledge of the material contained within *Intermediate Emergency Care.* Special projects include fill-in-the-blank and short-answer questions, matching exercises, etc.

EMERGENCY DRUG CARDS

The workbook contains alphabetized perforated 3" X 5" cards that present the emergency drug name, description, indications, contraindications, precautions, and dosage/route of the drugs included in the all-new appendix on emergency pharmacology. Detach the cards and use them as flash cards. Practice until you can give the correct route, dosage, indications, and contraindications for each drug.

ACKNOWLEDGMENTS

Special thanks must be given to those whose names do not appear on the cover of this workbook, yet without whom this effort would not have been possible. Names include Susan Katz, whose direction of the Brady Publishing line has brought new life into Emergency Medical Service education. Special thanks is given to Lois Berlowitz, who coordinated the editing process and assured the timely release of this workbook. Deb Parks is responsible for the development and copy editing that has made this document readable and more "englishly" correct. Finally, Craig N. Story, NREMT-P from Winter Haven, Florida, and Ed Kuvlesky, NREMT-P from Indian County, Florida, reviewed this workbook to ensure accuracy. Thank you all.

SPECIAL NOTE

The authors understand that there are constant changes in the knowledge and skills that we call emergency medical service. To that end, we have included a form at the end of the workbook. It is designed to record any comments, concerns, or corrections that you have regarding *Intermediate Emergency Care* or this workbook. Please record those comments and mail them to the address found on the form. We are interested in your comments and suggestions. Comments will be used to improve any subsequent printing or edition.

GUIDELINES TO BETTER TEST-TAKING

The knowledge you will gain from reading the textbook, completing the exercises in the workbook, listening to discussions in your EMT-Intermediate class, and participating in your clinical and field experience will prepare you to care for patients who are seriously ill or injured. However, before you can practice these skills, you will have to pass several classroom written exams and your state's certification exam. Your performance is not only dependent on your knowledge but also on your ability to answer test questions correctly. The following guidelines are designed to help improve your test performance and better reflect your knowledge of prehospital care.

1. Relax and be calm during the test.

A test is designed to measure what you have learned and to tell you and your instructor how well you are doing. An exam is not designed to intimidate you. Consider it a challenge and just try to do your best. Get plenty of sleep prior to the examination. Avoid coffee or other stimulants for a few hours before the exam. Be prepared, but relaxed.

Reread the text chapters, review the objectives in the workbook, and review your class notes. It might be helpful to work with one or two other students and ask each other questions. This type of practice helps everyone better understand the knowledge presented during your EMT-Intermediate training.

2. Read the questions carefully.

Read each word of the question slowly. Words such as <u>except</u> or <u>not</u> may change the entire meaning of the question. If you miss them, you may answer the question incorrectly even though you know the right answer.

Example
The art and science aspects of emergency medical services involve all of the following <u>except</u>
A. sincerity and compassion.
B. respect for human dignity.
C. placing patient care before personal safety.
D. delivery of sophisticated emergency medical care.
E. none of the above
The correct answer is C unless you miss the <u>except</u>.

3. Read each answer carefully.

Read each and every answer carefully. While the first answer may be absolutely correct, so may the rest, thus the best answer might be "all of the above."

Example
Indirect medical control is considered to be
A. treatment protocols.
B. training and education.
C. quality assurance.
D. chart review
E. all of the above
While answers A, B, C, and D are correct, the best and only acceptable answer is E, "all of the above."

4. Delay answering questions you don't understand and look for clues in the rest of the test.

When a question seems confusing or you don't know the answer, note it on your answer sheet and come back to it later. This will ensure that you have time to complete the test. You will also find that other questions in the test may give you hints to the one you've skipped over. It will also prevent you from being frustrated with an early question and have it affect your performance.

Example

Upon successful completion of a course of training as an EMT-Intermediate, most states will

A. certify you. (correct)

B. license you.

C. register you.

D. recognize you an an EMT-Intermediate.

E. issue you a permit.

Another question, later in the exam, may suggest the right answer.

The action of one state recognizing the certification of another is called

A. reciprocity. (correct)

B. national registration.

C. licensure.

D. registration.

E. extended practice.

5. **Answer all questions.**

Even if you do not know the right answers, do not leave a question blank. A blank question is always wrong, while a guess might be correct. If you can eliminate some of the answers, do so. It will increase the chances of a correct guess.

Example

When an EMT-Intermediate is called by the patient (through the dispatcher) to the scene of a medical emergency, the medical control physician has established a physician/patient relationship.

A. True

B. False

A True/False question gives you a 50% chance of a correct guess.

The hospital health professional responsible for sorting patients as they arrive at the emergency department is usually the

A. emergency physician.

B. ward clerk.

C. emergency nurse.

D. trauma surgeon.

E. A and C (correct)

A multiple-choice question with five answers gives a 20% chance of a correct guess. If you can eliminate one or more incorrect answers, you increase your odds of a correct guess to 25%, 33%, and so on. An unanswered question has a 0% chance of being correct.

Just before turning in your answer sheet, check to be sure you have not left any items blank.

CHAPTER 1

ROLES AND RESPONSIBILITIES OF THE EMT-INTERMEDIATE

REVIEW OF CHAPTER 1 OBJECTIVES

With each chapter of the workbook, we will identify the objectives and the important elements they describe. You should review them and refer to the pages listed if the elements are not clear.

After reading this chapter, you should be able to do the following:

Changes in the Field

1. Define the role of the EMT-Intermediate. *pp. 4–5*

Provides competent medical care

Provides emotional support for the patient

Concentrates on the care and well-being of the patient

Provides care to those who may not appreciate the service

2. Identify and describe those activities performed by an EMT-Intermediate in the field. *p. 9*

All the skills of the basic EMT

Advanced level assessment

Initiation of IVs

Advanced airway maneuvers, including endotracheal intubation

Care of the shock patient, including the PASG

In some systems, early defibrillation, intravenous glucose, etc.

Professional Ethics

3. Define and give examples of professional ethics. *pp. 9–12*

Rules or standards of conduct primarily for the benefit of the patient

Not laws, but standards for honorable behavior

A responsibility to the patient, society, health-care professionals, and the EMS profession

4. Describe the difference between ethical and legal requirements. *pp. 9–10*

Legal guidelines—an obligation to provide for the physical well-being of the patient

Ethical principals—an obligation to care for the patient's emotional well-being

Professionalism

5. Define and give examples of behavior that characterizes the health-care professional. *pp. 12–13*

Professionalism—conduct or qualities that characterize a practitioner in a particular field or occupation

A health-care professional will:

Place the patient first

Master and practice skills

Respond to emergency calls rapidly

Pursue continuing education

Prepare for response, maintaining vehicle, equipment, and personal mental fitness

Develop respect for other health-care and public-safety personnel

Focus on scene, rescuer, and patient safety rather than heroics

Role of the EMT-Intermediate

6. List the duties of the EMT-Intermediate in preparation for handling emergency medical responses. *pp. 14–15*

Keeps physically fit

Becomes familiar with system policies and procedures, communications, equipment, geography, and support agencies

Develops personal attributes of self-confidence, credibility, inner strength, self-control, leadership, and willingness to accept responsibility

7. List the duties of the EMT-Intermediate during an emergency response. *pp. 15–16*

Drives responsibly

Surveys the scene, calls for needed assistance, and assures scene and crew safety

Conducts patient assessment and assigns care priorities

Provides basic and advanced emergency medical care based on local protocols

Assesses the results of care

Communicates with team members and medical command

Directs transport of the patient to the appropriate medical facility

Maintains rapport with the patient and public-safety and hospital personnel

8. List the duties of the EMT-Intermediate after an emergency response. *pp. 16–17*

Accurately and objectively documents all elements of the response

Restocks the ambulance and assures that all equipment is clean and operational

Reviews the call with team members

Post-Graduate Responsibilities

9. List the post-graduation responsibilities of the EMT-Intermediate. *pp. 17–20*

Obtains and maintains licensure or certification

Maintains knowledge and skills

Updates knowledge and skills

Educates the public in First Aid, CPR, etc.

10. Distinguish among certification, licensure, and reciprocity. *p. 17*

Certification—recognition that an individual has met a standard of performance

Licensure—granting of permission to engage in an occupation

Reciprocity—granting of certification or licensure for comparable certification or licensure by another agency

11. State the benefits and responsibilities of continuing education for the EMT-Intermediate. *pp. 17–19*

Maintains initial skills and knowledge

Teaches new skills and knowledge

12. State the major purposes of a national organization. *p. 19*

Shares ideas and concerns

Speaks with a unified voice to the issues facing Emergency Medical Service

Provides continuing education (newsletters and conferences)

13. List some national organizations for EMS providers. *p. 19*

National Association of Emergency Medical Technicians

National Association of Flight Paramedics

National Association of Search and Rescue

National Council of State EMS Training Coordinators

National Association of State EMS Directors

National Association of EMS Physicians

14. State the major purposes of the National Registry of Emergency Medical Technicians. *p. 19*

Provides national testing of EMT-Basic, EMT-Intermediate, and EMT-Paramedic

Establishes standards for re-registration

Provides basis for interstate reciprocity

15. Describe the major benefits of subscribing to professional journals. *p. 19*

Maintains knowledge of current EMS research

Pursues continuing education

Provides a vehicle for authorship

CASE STUDY REVIEW

As was mentioned in Intermediate Emergency Care, *it is important to review each call that you participate in as an EMT-Intermediate. Similarly, review the case studies preceding each chapter of this text. We will address the important points of scene survey, patient assessment, patient management, patient packaging, and transport.*

Reread the case study in Intermediate Emergency Care *and then read the discussion below.*

This case study depicts a two-patient trauma call with the opportunity to focus on several elements of your response as an EMT-Intermediate.

CHAPTER 1 CASE STUDY

MED-1, with Stephen and Lisa, responds to a drive-by shooting. During the approximately four-minute drive to the scene, Lisa and Stephen discuss their respective roles. They talk about the primary survey and review the signs and symptoms of developing shock. Lisa mentions that they should not approach the area until the police clear them to enter and they are sure the scene is secure.

Once the police wave MED-1 in, the two EMT-Intermediates are joined by EMTs. Lisa and Stephen then each take a shooting victim. Stephen finds a young male with two gunshot wounds. Although the primary survey detects no suggestion of shock, Stephen will carefully reassess vital signs and the elements of the primary assessment periodically to monitor his condition. The location of the abdominal wound worries Stephen because the liver is a vascular organ that can bleed profusely and rapidly induce shock. For now, his patient is stable. But Stephen orders the EMTs to prepare the PASG while he initiates two IVs, just in case the patient's condition changes. Stephen decides that the patient is a candidate for rapid transport directly to the trauma center.

Lisa's patient does not exhibit injuries as critical as Stephen's patient. The primary assessment reveals no reason for concern so her attention focuses on the thigh wound. Once the pulse, capillary refill, and motor and sensory function are found to be normal, Lisa bandages the thigh and takes vital signs. Lisa decides to initiate an IV en route to the hospital. Although this patient is stable, Lisa knows that vascular injuries to this area may cause extensive yet hidden hemorrhage. Pressure caused by tissue swelling and hemorrhage may interfere with circulation as well as damage nerves. She will watch this patient closely to assure that his condition does not deteriorate.

The care offered on this call is a good example of what will be expected of you as an

EMT-Intermediate. However, not all the roles and responsibilities of an EMT- Intermediate are apparent. Lisa and Stephen have met the requirements of their state and are certified or licensed as EMT-Intermediates. Prior to this call, they assured their ambulance was clean, well maintained, and equipped with the needed supplies and equipment. Their dress is neat and clean, and their manner is professional. Most importantly, Lisa and Stephen take pride in what they do and take special care to meet not only the emergency care of the two patients' needs but their emotional needs as well. The actions of Stephen and Lisa will be remembered by the two patients and the bystanders at this incident for a long time to come.

CONTENT SELF-EVALUATION

Each of the chapters within this workbook includes a short content review. The questions are designed to test your ability to remember what you read. You can find the answers to the questions at the back of this workbook. If you answer any questions incorrectly, review the appropriate pages in the text.

MULTIPLE CHOICE

_____ **1.** The process by which an organization grants recognition that an individual has met its standards of performance is called
   A. licensure.
   B. certification.
   C. ethics.
   D. reciprocity.
   E. registration.

_____ **2.** The rules or standards governing the conduct of members of a particular group or profession are called
   A. ethics.
   B. morals.
   C. licensure.
   D. certification.
   E. registration.

_____ **3.** Since EMS is a science, EMT-Intermediates seldom face moral dilemmas.
   A. True
   B. False

_____ **4.** One of the greatest impacts upon the public's feelings toward the EMS system came from the television program *Emergency*. Which of the following are aspects of that program's presentation of EMS personnel?
   A. clean-cut
   B. respond promptly
   C. calm under stress
   D. skillful and compassionate
   E. all of the above

_____ **5.** The art and science aspects of emergency medical services involve all of the following except
   A. sincerity and compassion.
   B. respect for human dignity.
   C. placing patient care before personal safety.
   D. delivery of sophisticated emergency medical care.
   E. scene security.

_____ **6.** As members of the allied health professions, EMT-Intermediates must recognize a responsibility to
   A. their patients.
   B. society.
   C. other health professionals.
   D. themselves.
   E. all of the above

_____ **7.** The organization responsible for testing the various levels of EMTs on a national level is the
   A. National Association of EMTs.
   B. National Registry of EMTs.
   C. National Association of Search and Rescue.
   D. National Association of EMS Physicians.
   E. State Board of Health.

8. Accepting standards established by another agency or state is called
A. licensure.
B. certification.
C. reciprocity.
D. registration.
E. diversification.

9. The EMT-Intermediate has a responsibility to become familiar with support services in his or her area.
A. True
B. False

10. The ambulance run report should include which of the following?
A. accurate and complete documentation
B. clear and concise opinions
C. objectively recorded observations
D. A and C
E. A and B

11. Upon successful completion of a course of training as an EMT-Intermediate, most states will
A. certify you.
B. license you.
C. register you.
D. recognize you as an EMT-Intermediate.
E. issue you a permit.

12. After a call, an EMT-Intermediate is responsible for
A. restocking the ambulance.
B. completing the run report.
C. ensuring that team members are not affected by stress.
D. reviewing the call with team members.
E. all of the above

13. Continuing education is intended to
A. maintain an EMT-Intermediate's initial knowledge.
B. address didactic knowledge only.
C. broaden an EMT-Intermediate's knowledge.
D. A and C.
E. none of the above

14. Professional journals provide an EMT-Intermediate with
A. an opportunity to write and publish articles.
B. a source of continuing education material.
C. information on new procedures for the field.
D. all of the above.
E. none of the above.

15. The EMT-Intermediate will most probably spend more time preparing to perform his or her duties (cleaning and restocking the ambulance, reading and attending continuing education sessions, documenting the last call, etc.) than responding to emergency medical calls.
A. True
B. False

DESCRIPTION

16. List at least three responsibilities of the EMT-Intermediate in preparation for an EMS response.

_____

_____

_____

17. List at least five responsibilities of the EMT-Intermediate during the emergency response.

_____

_____

_____

_____

_____

_____

18. Identify at least five attributes of leadership that an EMT-Intermediate should have.

_____

_____

_____

_____

_____

_____

19. Describe the expectations the public has of the EMS system because of popular television programs depicting EMS personnel at work.

_____

_____

_____

_____

_____

_____

20. List at least three possibilities for continuing education that an EMT-Intermediate might pursue.

_____

_____

_____

_____

_____

_____

SPECIAL PROJECT

Write to the National Registry of EMTs and ask for brochures. Consider joining the organization at this time. The address can be found in the Answer Key at the back of this workbook.

CHAPTER 2

EMERGENCY MEDICAL SERVICES SYSTEMS

REVIEW OF CHAPTER 2 OBJECTIVES

After reading this chapter, you should be able to do the following:

History of EMS System Development

1. List and define the components of an EMS system. *pp. 24–27*

Prehospital Component

Bystanders who recognize the emergency

Lay persons trained in CPR and first aid

First Responders

EMT-Basics

EMT-Intermediates

EMT-Paramedics

Hospital Component

Emergency Physicians

Emergency Nurses

Specialty Physicians (e.g., trauma surgeons and cardiologists)

2. Describe the development of the EMS system in the United States. *pp. 27–29*

Accidental Death and Disability: The Neglected Disease of Modern Society—described the poor state of prehospital care and suggested guidelines for the development of EMS systems

1966 Highway Safety Act—forced states to develop EMS systems

1973 Emergency Medical Services System Act—established regional EMS systems

1981 Consolidated Omnibus Budget Reconciliation Act (COBRA)—wiped out federal funding of EMS, except block grants administered by the Department of Transportation

The System Approach

3. Explain the oversight duties of an EMS administrative agency. *p. 29*

Regional and Municipal Systems

Designate who may function within the system

Develop policies consistent with state requirements

Develop quality assurance or improvement programs

State Systems

Allocate funds to regional systems

Enact legislation concerning the prehospital practice of medicine

License or certify field providers

Enforce state regulations

Appoint regional advisory councils

4. Discuss the responsibilities of the physician medical director regarding direct (on-line) and indirect (off-line) medical control. *pp. 30–33*

General Responsibilities

Delegates authority to practice medicine in the prehospital setting

Remains responsible for patient care regardless of whether medical control is direct or indirect

Direct

Directs communication with medical control physician

Responsible for patient-delegate care

Involves EMT/physician interaction

Indirect

Training and continuing education

Medical protocols (non-interaction)

  Triage

  Treatment

  Transport

  Transfer

Medical audit/chart review/quality assurance

5. Define and compare standing orders and protocols as used in prehospital care. *pp. 31–33*

Protocols—policies and procedures for all components of an EMS system

Standing orders—field-care interventions that are completed before contacting the direct medical control physician

6. Explain public involvement in an EMS system, including system access, recognition of an emergency, and initiation of basic life support. *pp. 33–34*

The public should be:

  Offered training and information to increase their knowledge of system entry—9-1-1, single number, or multi-number entry

  Encouraged to take lay-person training in First Aid and CPR

7. Identify the components of an effective medical and organizational communications system. *pp. 35–39*

Citizen access

Single control center

Organizational communications capabilities

Medical communications capabilities

Hardware (radios, towers, pagers, etc.)

Software (frequencies, protocols, communications plans)

8. Describe the components of emergency medical dispatching. *pp. 38–39*

System status management—dynamic use of resources to best meet the needs of the service area and ambulance crews

Interrogation guidelines—used to ensure that the appropriate information is gathered from the caller

Response protocols—used to guide the dispatcher in matching the caller's information with the most appropriate unit(s) and personnel for the patient's need

Pre-arrival instructions—used to communicate care instructions to the caller, assisting him or her in providing patient care

Dispatcher training—assures both medical and technical preparation for their role

9. Explain the importance of quality evaluation in EMS. *pp. 31–41*

Ensures proper training

Teaches a high regard for human dignity and a passion for excellence

Emphasizes that certification marks the beginning—not the end—of education

10. Explain the coordination of patient transfer with ground and air transport services. *p. 43*

Patient transport protocols should:

Take into account the nature of the patient's problem, the severity of the patient's condition, the distance to the various facilities, and the specialty services of the various hospitals

Make efficient use of BLS, ALS, and aeromedical services

11. Discuss the similarities and differences between quality assurance and quality improvement programs. *pp. 44–46*

Quality assurance—programs that objectively identify problems and continuously monitor the quality of an EMS system or service

Quality improvement—programs that focus on the perceptions of the patient ("the customer") as well as the items evaluated by the quality assurance programs

12. Discuss the value of research in EMS. *pp. 46–47*

Determines which care procedures/equipment benefit the patient

Determines benefit/risk ratio for procedures

Determines cost/benefit of sophisticated EMS interventions

Determines if immediate transport or scene care is appropriate

13. Describe the categorization of receiving facilities, and explain how the coordination of resources is attained. *pp. 47–48*

Categorization—allows transportation of patients to appropriate special-service facilities—i.e., burn, trauma, pediatric, perinatal, cardiac, spinal, psychiatric, or poison control centers

Coordination—attained through a central hospital so that the needs of a particular patient are met by the regional system

14. List the components of mutual aid and mass-casualty planning. *pp. 48–49*

Mutual aid agreements

Mass-casualty plans

Coordinated central management agency

Frequent drills

CASE STUDY REVIEW

Reread the case study in Intermediate Emergency Care, *and then read the discussion below.*

This case study is an overview of the Emergency Medical Services System with a focus on system entry, the contributions that trained bystanders can provide, and the tiered response system.

CHAPTER 2 CASE STUDY

The call described by this case study is all too typical in rural America. Therefore, you may soon find yourself in the position of the two EMT-Intermediates who answered this call. You will be asked to oversee the care of your patients, make some very important decisions, and be part of the Emergency Medical Services system. To fulfill this role, you must understand the system in which you work as well as the personnel and administrative structures that coordinate activity within the system.

The response described here is a tiered response. The two EMTs arrive as first responders and begin the formal emergency medical care at the scene. The second tier of response is the fire department EMT-Intermediates who quickly transition to medical care leadership roles over the two patients. This transition takes place as a smooth exchange starting with a quick report of findings from the EMTs to the EMT-Intermediates. The EMT-Intermediates ask any needed questions and then begin to direct further care.

One decision that must be made deals with patient condition. The seriousness of the accident suggests the need for prompt transport. However, the closest ambulance is at a community hospital about 30 miles away. So the EMT-Intermediates summon a helicopter instead. The helicopter will greatly reduce travel time. It will also bring more advanced life support to the patient. The services of a nurse, paramedic, and physician will be helpful in aggressively treating the viable patient described in the scenario.

At this point, the EMT-Intermediates begin to practice medicine under the direction of the medical control physician (on-line or direct medical control) and under the physician's license. That permission can only be extended through prearranged permission to practice called protocols (off-line or indirect medical control) or through direct physician contact, as occurs in the case study. In either situation, this ability to provide invasive medical procedures is the result of a sophisticated system of physicians and prehospital and hospital personnel. This system determines, in advance, what you as an EMT-Intermediate can do and under what circumstances. The system will also determine under what circumstances you can provide care before or only after direct contact with a physician.

After the EMT-Intermediates complete the call, it will be reviewed by the system quality improvement committee. Members will examine how the system responded to the needs of the two patients. They will examine the adherence to protocols, the interaction with medical control, the appropriateness of helicopter utilization, the evaluation of the patient's condition at the scene, and the perceptions from bystanders, care providers, and the surviving patient. This information will be used to determine how well the system functioned and will identify any improvements that could be made. Infrequently, the quality improvement committee directs remediation to individual care providers.

CONTENT SELF-EVALUATION

MULTIPLE CHOICE

_____ 1. The system that makes use of several levels of responding emergency medical services personnel—the First Responder, EMT, and Paramedic—is called
A. the tiered response system.
B. a multifaceted system.
C. an advanced life support system.
D. a fail-safe system.
E. volunteer-supplemented system.

_____ 2. All prehospital medical care provided by the EMT-Intermediate is considered an extension of the medical director's license.
A. True
B. False

_____ 3. The hospital health professional responsible for sorting patients as they arrive at the emergency department is usually the
A. floor nurse.
B. ward clerk.
C. emergency nurse.
D. trauma surgeon.
E. surgical assistant.

_____ 4. Medical control provided by on-line radio contact between the EMT-Intermediate and the medical control physician is known as
A. protocol.
B. direct.
C. indirect.
D. intrinsic.
E. extrinsic.

_____ **5.** When an EMT-Intermediate is called by the patient (through the dispatcher) to the scene of a medical emergency, the medical control physician has established a physician/patient relationship.
 A. True
 B. False

_____ **6.** The physician who called for EMT-Intermediates to transport his or her patient, without accompanying the patient, remains in charge and responsible for the care provided to the patient until the patient is attended by another physician in the emergency department.
 A. True
 B. False

_____ **7.** Indirect medical control includes
 A. treatment protocols.
 B. training and education.
 C. quality assurance.
 D. chart review.
 E. all of the above

_____ **8.** Protocols standardize field procedures. They should not allow the EMT-Intermediate flexibility to improvise nor adapt to special circumstances.
 A. True
 B. False

_____ **9.** The device that may in the future be used by the first responder or bystander to improve significantly the survival rates of patients in cardiac arrest is the
 A. transcutaneous pacemaker.
 B. esophageal obturator airway.
 C. automatic external defibrillator.
 D. pulse oximeter.
 E. glucometer.

_____ **10.** The dispatch system that reduces response time by locating ambulances based upon projected call volume is called
 A. priority dispatching.
 B. system status management.
 C. interrogation protocols.
 D. medical direction.
 E. pre-planned dispatching.

_____ **11.** The dispatch system that interrogates the caller, prioritizes symptoms, selects the appropriate response, and provides the caller with life-saving instructions is called
 A. priority dispatching.
 B. system status management.
 C. interrogation protocols.
 D. medical direction.
 E. simplex dispatching.

_____ **12.** The ideal EMS dispatch system includes
 A. caller interrogation protocols.
 B. pre-determined response configurations and system status management.
 C. pre-arrival instructions for caller and strong medical control.
 D. A and C
 E. all of the above

_____ **13.** Quality assurance and quality improvement programs look at
 A. response times.
 B. adherence to protocols.
 C. patient survival.
 D. customer perceptions.
 E. all of the above

_____ **14.** Many protocols and procedures that EMT-Intermediates use today have evolved without clinical evidence of their usefulness, safety, or benefit to the patient.
 A. True
 B. False

_____ **15.** Quality improvement programs differ from quality assurance programs in that quality improvement also looks at
A. customer satisfaction.
B. dispatch procedures.
C. quality of care.
D. mortality and morbidity.
E. none of the above

_____ **16.** An example of hospital categorization is
A. a Burn Center.
B. a Trauma Center.
C. a Perinatal Center.
D. a Cardiac Center.
E. all of the above

_____ **17.** EMS system funding can come from
A. tax subsidies.
B. Medicare, Medicaid.
C. subscription plans.
D. user fees.
E. all of the above

_____ **18.** The elements of a mass-casualty plan should include
A. closely defined geographical boundaries.
B. a flexible communication system.
C. a central management structure
D. B and C
E. all of the above

_____ **19.** EMS systems are designed with the patient as the highest priority. They begin with a strong administrative agency that structures the system around the patient's needs and grants the medical director ultimate authority in all issues of patient care.
A. True
B. False

SEQUENCING

20. Place the steps below in the order in which they would occur in a research project. Number the first step 1, the second step 2, and so on.

_____ **A.** develop a hypothesis or question to be asked

_____ **B.** prepare a paper for a magazine

_____ **C.** collect and analyze data

_____ **D.** search the literature

DESCRIPTION

21. Identify the purpose of each of the four types of protocols.

Triage: (at least 1)

_____

Treatment: (at least 2)

_____

_____

Transport: (at least 2)

_____

_____

Transfer: (at least 1)

_____

22. What skills are associated with these levels of Emergency Medical Services certification?

EMT-Basic: (at least 5)

_____

_____

_____

_____

_____

EMT-Intermediate: (at least 2)

_____

_____

EMT-Paramedic: (at least 4)

_____

_____

_____

_____

23. Identify and describe the four elements of the priority dispatch system.

A. _____

_____

_____

B. _____

_____

_____

C. _____

_____

_____

D. _____

_____

_____

SPECIAL PROJECT

Using your knowledge of basic life support, design a research project that investigates the accuracy of blood pressure determination among EMTs.

Hypothesis: Write a hypothesis (a statement that defines what you are trying to prove or disprove).

Literature review: Where would you look for information? (search of the literature: magazines, journals, textbooks, etc.)

Study methods: Explain how you would test your hypothesis. (description of what you would do to verify your hypothesis: field study, clinical trial, etc.)

Conclusion: Explain the results of the research, and how it supports or rejects your hypothesis. (completed only when the results of the research are known)

CHAPTER 3

MEDICAL-LEGAL CONSIDERATIONS OF EMERGENCY CARE

REVIEW OF CHAPTER 3 OBJECTIVES

After reading this chapter, you should be able to do the following:

Legal Principles

1. Describe the two general categories of law in the United States and give examples of each. pp. 54–55

Criminal law—addresses crime and punishment and involves legal action against an individual by the state
Examples: homicide and rape

Civil law—deals with noncriminal matters
Examples: contract disputes, divorce, torts

2. Define the following terms. pp. 55–65

Tort—deals with civil wrongs committed by one individual against another, such as a malpractice suit

Assault—any action that places a person in fear of immediate bodily harm

False imprisonment—intentional and unjustifiable detention of a person against his or her will

Duty to act—the obligation to respond to a situation

Libel—act of injuring someone's name or character by false or malicious writing

Negligence—deviation from accepted standard of care

Battery—act of unlawfully touching another person without his or her consent

Abandonment—termination of a health care provider-patient relationship without assurance that equal or greater care will continue

Slander—act of injuring someone's name or character by false or malicious spoken words

Laws Affecting EMS

3. Discuss the medical practice act and its implications in prehospital care. p. 56

Medical practice act—state legislation that sets the standards for the practice of medicine

Implications—allows the EMT-Intermediate to perform as an agent under the license of a physician

4. Explain what is meant by the term "delegation of authority." p. 56

The EMT-Intermediate functions as the agent of medical control, or an authorized physician

5. Describe the purpose and limitations of Good Samaritan Laws. pp. 56–57

Purpose—provide protection against negligence proceedings for those who render care at an emergency scene without compensation, offer their services in good faith, and are not negligent

Limitations—the constitutionality of Good Samaritan Laws is being challenged

6. Explain the need to know state motor vehicle laws that apply to emergency vehicles. *p. 57*

Provisions extend special privileges and place certain responsibilities on the operator of an authorized emergency vehicle

7. Explain the purpose of a "Living Will," "Durable Power of Attorney for Health Care," and a "Do Not Resuscitate" order. *pp. 58–59*

Living Will—legal document by which a patient specifies the kinds of medical treatment he or she wishes to receive in cases of serious injury or illness

Durable Power of Attorney for Health Care—legal document that designates another person to make health-care decisions for a patient

Do Not Resuscitate order—order written by a physician directing that resuscitation should be withheld; when in doubt of a DNR's authenticity, resuscitation should be provided

Standard of Care

8. Discuss the concept of "standard of care" as it applies to prehospital care. *p. 60*

Standard against which an EMT-Intermediate will be judged to determine negligence

Care a similarly trained and experienced EMT-Intermediate would be expected to provide under similar circumstances

9. List and define the four components required to prove negligence in a malpractice proceeding. *p. 60*

Duty to act—that an EMT-Intermediate had a legal obligation to care for a patient

Breach of Duty—that the EMT-Intermediate failed to meet the expected standard of care

Damages—that the EMT-Intermediate caused injury or harm to the patient

Proximate cause—that actions taken by the EMT-Intermediate were the direct cause of harm experienced by the patient

10. Discuss the concept of *res ipsa loquitur.* *pp. 60–61*

Literal meaning—"the thing speaks for itself"

Legal meaning—that the damages would not have occurred in the absence of somebody's negligence; that the instruments of damage were under the defendant's control at all times; that the patient did nothing to contribute to his or her injury

11. Define the term "informed consent," and relate it to the practice of prehospital emergency care. *p. 61*

Informed consent—consent obtained only after the patient understands the nature, extent, and potential risks of treatment; required prior to beginning prehospital care

Required for prehospital care to begin legally

12. Discuss the following types of consent: *p. 62*

Expressed consent—occurs when a patient verbally, nonverbally, or in writing, gives permission to receive medical treatment

Implied consent—presumed from a patient who is unable to provide informed consent either due to inability to communicate or mental impairment

Non-voluntary consent—consent for treatment issued by the court and against the patient's wishes

13. Define assault and battery, and give examples of each. *pp. 64–65*

Assault—any action that places a person in immediate fear of bodily harm
Example: approaching a patient with a catheter to start an IV without permission to treat

Battery—act of touching a person without his or her consent
Example: attempting to apply a traction splint without first gaining the patient's permission

Medical Liability Protection

14. Discuss the importance of the medical record. *p. 66*

　Permanent record of all actions, procedures, and medications administered during a call

　May be the only record of what happened during a later legal proceeding

15. List several methods of protecting yourself from malpractice liability. *p. 66*

　Practice good prehospital care

　Provide care for the patient as you would wish to be cared for

　Document all runs completely and appropriately

　Purchase and maintain malpractice insurance

CASE STUDY REVIEW

Reread the case study in Intermediate Emergency Care *and then read the discussion below.*

This call represents a realistic emergency medical response that has many elements of interest from a medical-legal point of view. It identifies a number of situations that may put you, as an EMT-Intermediate, at risk of malpractice if you do not employ proper legal principles.

CHAPTER 3 CASE STUDY

En route to the scene, the EMT-Intermediates of Ambulance 6 prepare for a full cardiac arrest. They ready and check the oxygen, airway equipment, and suction. They also review their roles in the impending resuscitation and their system's cardiac arrest protocols. For example, they might plan to initiate resuscitation by invoking implied consent. The patient will be unable otherwise to give consent, and hence they assume the patient would consent if indeed he could.

　Upon arrival, EMT-Intermediates observe that the patient has respiratory problems, rather than a cardiac arrest. They also face family members with different requests about how to proceed. The two EMTs must sort out the legalities while attending to the patient's needs. The daughter requests that he be allowed to die, while the patient's wife asks for aggressive resuscitation. The only circumstance where an EMT-Intermediate would not resuscitate is when they find a valid "Do Not Resuscitate" order. Such an order is prescribed by state law and varies across the nation. When in doubt, an EMS team should provide care.

　In this case, someone requested an ambulance—a clear call for help. Secondly, the spouse of the patient requests care. Further, a "Do Not Resuscitate" order is not available. The EMT-Intermediates' decision to resuscitate this patient is appropriate.

　Another legal consideration in this scenario is patient consent. The EMT-Intermediate assessing the patient must determine the patient's level of consciousness and ability to give consent. If the patient is found to be alert, the EMT-Intermediate must explain what care will be provided and give the patient the opportunity to decline such care. If the patient is unresponsive, consent is implied. If the patient then becomes conscious and alert, he may refuse care and the crew of Ambulance 6 would have to cease care and explain the possible consequences of halting care (withdrawal of consent). It would also be necessary to have the patient sign a written release form and have it witnessed by someone other than the ambulance crew.

　In this case, the EMT-Intermediates placed an endotracheal tube, which is an invasive advanced life support procedure. Such a procedure is permitted only through delegation of authority from the medical control physician to the prehospital care provider. They may employ such a procedure via a standing order or after direct communication with the physician via radio. Failure to get the appropriate permission for the procedure or performing advanced skills beyond the local protocol may expose the care providers to charges of practicing medicine without a license.

　After this call, the EMT-Intermediates will document the call on the run report. They must be accurate and keep all information confidential. The use of slang, derogatory labels, or subjective statements in the report may expose the care providers to charges of libel—the act of injuring a person's character or reputation by malicious or false writings. The report may also be examined in a court of law to determine what care was given and if it was appropriate. Poor documentation may call into question the quality of care given. Complete, accurate, and appropriate documentation will substantiate complete, accurate, and appropriate care.

To extend this case, consider this scenario:

Both the EMT-Intermediates attending this patient have their own malpractice insurance. The company they work for has a blanket policy covering a potential law suit. However, when they investigated the coverage the EMTs found that individuals were not well covered. Also, the policy did not cover the EMT-Intermediates while off duty or while working for the rural services in which they volunteer. Their personal malpractice insurance is inexpensive and affords them some peace of mind. You might do well by investigating your own coverage.

CONTENT SELF-EVALUATION

MULTIPLE CHOICE

_____ **1.** The principle allowing an EMT-Intermediate to function in the field under the auspices and license of a physician is called
- **A.** res ipsa loquitur.
- **B.** medical control.
- **C.** the Good Samaritan principle.
- **D.** delegation of authority.
- **E.** none of the above

_____ **2.** An EMT-Intermediate may become involved in the legal system because he or she will be called
- **A.** as a witness in a criminal offense.
- **B.** to testify in a civil matter.
- **C.** to defend himself or herself in a malpractice suit.
- **D.** to testify in a contract dispute.
- **E.** all of the above

_____ **3.** The Good Samaritan Law was designed to protect EMS personnel against legal liability resulting from negligent care.
- **A.** True
- **B.** False

_____ **4.** Generally, which circumstances require an EMT-Intermediate to report an incident to law enforcement officials?
- **A.** child or elderly abuse
- **B.** rape or sexual abuse
- **C.** a shooting
- **D.** physical assault
- **E.** all of the above

_____ **5.** *You respond to a home where a patient has a "do not resuscitate" order.* You are obligated to provide Advanced Life Support to the limit of your training and ability.
- **A.** True
- **B.** False

_____ **6.** The principle of providing the same level of treatment as any other similarly trained individual would provide in a similar situation is called
- **A.** negligence.
- **B.** standard of care.
- **C.** duty to act.
- **D.** an act of omission.
- **E.** proximate cause.

_____ **7.** In a malpractice suit, the plaintiff must prove all of the following except
- **A.** the EMT-Intermediate had a duty to act.
- **B.** the party was damaged or injured.
- **C.** the EMT-Intermediate failed to meet the standard of care.
- **D.** actions by the EMT-Intermediate caused some of the damages.
- **E.** the party was slandered.

_____ **8.** Caring for a patient without obtaining the proper consent is grounds for charges of
- **A.** assault and battery.
- **B.** malpractice.
- **C.** negligence.
- **D.** *res ipsa loquitur.*
- **E.** B and C

_____ **9.** Once a patient has given consent for care, he or she cannot refuse further care until evaluated by a physician.
- **A.** True
- **B.** False

_____ **10.** The permission to provide care after a patient understands the benefits and risks of treatment is called
- **A.** the patient's right to know.
- **B.** informed consent.
- **C.** duty to act.
- **D.** implied consent.
- **E.** none of the above

_____ **11.** A patient's refusal to receive care and/or be transported should be
- **A.** recorded in the run report.
- **B.** signed by the patient.
- **C.** witnessed by someone other than the EMS crew.
- **D.** all of the above
- **E.** B and C only

_____ **12.** Recording false and malicious information on a patient's run report might subject an EMT-Intermediate to legal action because of
- **A.** libel.
- **B.** medical control policy violation.
- **C.** malpractice.
- **D.** slander.
- **E.** violation of a medical practice act.

DESCRIPTION

13. Compare and contrast negligence and *res ipsa loquitur* as they apply to the EMT-Intermediate.

_____

_____

_____

_____

_____

_____

14. List three potential patient conditions in which care can be given even though patient consent cannot be obtained.

_____

_____

_____

_____

15. Reread the case study for this chapter, and briefly record the essential information that should be written in the narrative run report.

_____

_____

_____

_____

_____

SPECIAL PROJECT

List your state's requirements for licensure of an EMT-Intermediate ambulance service.

Personnel Requirements:

How many persons must respond with the ambulance?

What training must they have?

Vehicle Requirements:

What type of vehicle is required?

Equipment Requirements:

What emergency care equipment is required?

What radio equipment is required?

CHAPTER 4

MEDICAL TERMINOLOGY

REVIEW OF CHAPTER 4 OBJECTIVES

After reading this chapter, you should be able to do the following:

Medical Dictionary

1. Locate at least six medical terms in a medical dictionary. p. 72

Medical dictionaries provide:

Essential tools for practicing EMT-Intermediates

Opportunities to investigate the meanings of new terms and to confirm spellings for documentation

A way to communicate more professionally with physicians, nurses, and other health-care personnel

Medical Terminology

2. Identify common root words and define their meaning. pp. 73–77

Root word—conveys the essential meaning of a word; the word to which a suffix, prefix, or both is attached

3. Identify and define common prefixes and suffixes. pp. 77–81

Prefix—one or more syllables affixed to the beginning of a root word to modify its meaning

Suffix—one or more syllables affixed to the end of a root word to modify its meaning

4. Identify and determine the meaning of common medical terms. pp. 72–81

To define a medical term:

Identify the meaning of each word part

Check definitions in a medical dictionary

Abbreviations

5. Identify common medical abbreviations. pp. 81–87

Use of abbreviations:

Enhances efficiency in recording common signs, symptoms, and care procedures

Reduces the time and space needed to record this data on run reports

CASE STUDY REVIEW

Reread the case study in Intermediate Emergency Care and then read the narrative below.

This case study highlights the importance of medical terminology as you care for a patient and interact with the medical community.

CHAPTER 4 CASE STUDY

The crew of Ambulance 945 is presented with a rather typical trauma call. They survey the scene to reveal a patient who fell about 30 feet into an area of construction debris. Robert, the senior EMT-Intermediate, directs rescue personnel to remove some of the debris to assure scene safety and to facilitate patient assessment, care, and removal. Due to the height of the fall, this patient is a candidate for rapid transport to the closest trauma center. The primary assessment and initial stabilization will be accomplished and transport begun without delay.

Signs detected by Glen in the secondary survey reveal potential for internal injury. The tender abdomen suggests internal hemorrhage, and the unstable pelvis may reflect the cause. Pelvic fractures that cause instability frequently cause severe blood loss. Of additional concern is the paralysis of the lower extremities. Spine injury or the pelvic fracture may account for this finding.

The vital signs are within normal limits. The pulse rate is a bit high, an early sign of shock, though it may be caused by the patient's excitement or response to pain. The blood pressure is a bit low, which may reflect a healthy male or an early result of blood loss. As a result of the findings of the secondary survey, the mechanism of injury, and the vital signs, Robert and Glen start one IV with a large-bore catheter and lactated Ringer's solution. They gently apply a cervical collar, move the patient to the spine board while observing spinal precautions, and immobilize him.

As Ambulance 945 travels to the trauma center, Robert calls the medical control physician to give the patient report. During this short radio transmission, Robert must accurately communicate the circumstances that brought his patient into the emergency medical services system as well as the results of the primary and secondary assessments and vital signs determination. He must also communicate the care the crew has provided and request instructions for further care. To accomplish this, Robert uses the standard radio report format, as will be discussed in Chapter 5, and the appropriate medical terminology.

Robert's report is brief, yet it paints a clear picture of his findings. The mechanism of injury and chief complaint are communicated, as is the patient's pertinent medical history, including his allergies and previous medical problems. The vital signs and findings of the physical assessment are included, as are pertinent negative findings: no loss of consciousness and no incontinence. Finally, Robert provides a report of the care given and the estimated time of arrival.

Once at the Emergency Department, Robert and Glen will continue relaying information to the staff and the emergency physician. Their correct use of medical terminology, the language of medicine, will help them quickly and concisely inform the trauma center personnel of the patient's condition and his emergency needs. They will also document the events and findings of the call on the run report. They will use the appropriate terminology and medical abbreviations to provide a precise narrative.

MEDICAL TERM DISSECTION

Identify the meaning of the root word, prefix, and suffix for each of the medical terms listed below. (Not all terms have both prefixes and suffixes.)

Please note that some root words, prefixes, and suffixes can be used interchangeably.

	Prefix	Root	Suffix
1. myasthenia	_____	_____	_____
2. cephalgia	_____	_____	_____
3. percuss	_____	_____	_____
4. cyanosis	_____	_____	_____
5. hyperflexion	_____	_____	_____
6. pathology	_____	_____	_____
7. tachypnea	_____	_____	_____
8. rhinorrhea	_____	_____	_____
9. dysuria	_____	_____	_____
10. hypertrophy	_____	_____	_____
11. osteocyte	_____	_____	_____

12. hypoxemia _____ _____ _____

14. hepatomegaly _____ _____ _____

15. abduct _____ _____ _____

16. otoscope _____ _____ _____

17. perinatal _____ _____ _____

18. antecubital _____ _____ _____

19. dissect _____ _____ _____

20. epicardium _____ _____ _____

21. postpartum _____ _____ _____

22. intervertebral _____ _____ _____

23. neuroplasty _____ _____ _____

24. hemothorax _____ _____ _____

25. polyphagia _____ _____ _____

Identify the meaning of these common medical abbreviations.

26. abd. _____

27. ARDS _____

28. ASHD _____

29. AMA _____

30. BBB _____

31. b.i.d. _____

32. C/C _____

33. CHF _____

34. COPD _____

35. CSF _____

36. Dx _____

37. DPT _____

38. ETOH _____

39. fx _____

40. GSW _____

41. GU _____

42. Hct. _____

43. Hx _____

44. IPPB _____

45. JVD _____

46. MVA _____

47. NPO _____

48. PRN _____

49. pt. _____

50. Rx _____

51. S/S _____

52. S.O.B. _____

53. TKO _____

54. wt. _____

55. y.o. _____

SPECIAL PROJECT

Locate the following medical terms in a medical dictionary.

acromegaly	bathophobia	blastocyte
cathartic	cynanthropy	dipsomania
ergotherapy	hypoglossal	leukocytogenesis
monomorphic	prodromal	serotonin

CHAPTER 5
EMS COMMUNICATIONS

REVIEW OF CHAPTER 5 OBJECTIVES

After reading this chapter, you should be able to do the following:

EMS Communication Links

1. Describe the sequence of an EMS event. *pp. 93–94*

Occurrence—illness or injury that provides the need for the EMS response

Detection—recognition that there is a need for the EMS response

Notification and response—call to appropriate EMS personnel and direction of units to the scene

Treatment and preparation—phase in which the patient is assessed, managed, and prepared for transport

Transport and delivery—loading, transport, continuation of care, and the delivery of the patient to the emergency department

Preparation for the next event—cleaning and restocking of the ambulance, completion of paperwork, notification of EMS dispatch that the EMS unit is back in service

2. Describe the five communications phases of an EMS response. *pp. 94–97*

Notification—notification of an emergency situation by a citizen, municipal worker, etc.

Dispatch—alerting and sending the appropriate EMS personnel to the scene

Medical communications—transmission of the results of patient assessment to the medical command physician and a request for permission to employ care procedures

Hospital arrival—phase of communication in which an EMT-Intermediate verbally informs the medical control physician of what was found in the field, what care steps were offered, what results came of that care, and what was revealed by a pertinent patient history

In service—notification to the dispatcher that the unit has been restocked, cleaned, and is back in service

Communications Systems: Technical Aspects

3. Define the following terms: *pp. 97–103*

Base station—principal transmitter and receiver of an EMS system; located close to the antenna and is usually operated by a remote unit found in the dispatch center

Mobile two-way transmitter/receiver—vehicle mounted radio unit with a lower transmission power than the base station

Portable radio—hand-held radio unit with less power and range than the mobile radio

Repeater—radio base station modified to retransmit a radio broadcast so the area covered by the EMS system can be increased; normally located strategically within the service area and tied to the dispatch center by either a telephone or radio link

Voting—process by which the repeater station receiving the strongest incoming signal is chosen to rebroadcast that signal

Remote console—unit designed to control the base station from a location some distance away

Encoder—electronic device that generates unique signals or tones within a radio transmission; signals can be recognized by another radio's decoder

Decoder—electronic device that listens to radio transmissions and recognizes only those signals for which it is encoded

4. Describe the advantages of a repeater system over a nonrepeater system. *pp. 99–100*

Permits a communications network to be dependable over a large service area or through terrain that otherwise would limit communications

Often allows communications even though one tower may be inoperative

Offers greater assurance that weak transmissions from a mobile or portable unit will be heard

Radio Communications

5. List the two types of radio wave transmission. *pp. 102–103*

Amplitude modulation—modification of a radio transmission by varying the amplitude of the signal; referred to as AM; has a relatively poor quality of transmission, though its range is good

Frequency modulation—modification of a radio transmission by varying the frequency of the signal; referred to as FM; has very good quality of transmission, though its range is less than that of AM

6. Define the following terms: *pp. 103–104*

Hertz—number of cycles of electrical activity per second in a radio signal

Band—group of radio frequencies close together in the electromagnetic spectrum

Trunking—computer-assisted radio system that maximizes the use of available radio channels

Biotelemetry—process of transmitting physiological data, such as an electrocardiogram, usually by radio

Modulator—device that electronically transforms electrical energy into sound waves that may be transmitted

Demodulator—device that recognizes a specific modulated transmission and converts it back to electrical impulses

7. Describe the 10 "Med Channels" and their usage. *pp. 103–104*

Med Channels—ultra high frequency (UHF) channels designated as medical communications channels; duplex pairs designed for advanced life support service

Usage—channels one through eight are for paramedic/medical control communications; nine and ten are reserved for EMS dispatch

8. Describe the most common causes of interference in biotelemetry communications. *p. 104*

Muscle tremors, loose electrodes, 60 Hz interference (from other electrical sources)

Fluctuations in transmitter power

Transmission of voice and telemetry simultaneously

Equipment Maintenance

9. Discuss the importance of communications equipment maintenance. *p. 104*

Protects fragile, expensive equipment and ensures that it operates when needed

Proper maintenance requires:

> Regular cleaning
> Proper repair of malfunctions
> Frequent recharging of batteries
> Storage of spare batteries

Rules and Operating Procedures

10. Describe briefly the functions and responsibilities of the Federal Communications Commission. *p. 105*

The Federal Communications Commission is responsible for the overall operation and regulation of radio service. It approves equipment, allocates frequencies, licenses transmitters, licenses repair personnel, monitors the system, and spot-checks station records.

11. Define briefly the role of the EMS dispatcher. p. 106

    Responsible for gathering information from the caller

    Instructs the caller in limited first aid procedures

    Directs the appropriate resources (EMS, fire department, police, etc.) to the right location

    Monitors the response to a call by the responding units

    Monitors general radio communications

12. Describe how the information necessary to initiate an EMS response is obtained. pp. 106–107

    Access of the EMS system by the victim, a relative or friend of the victim, a bystander, or another member of the public safety service system, like a police officer

    Interrogation of the caller by the dispatcher to determine the nature of the call, the exact location, and any other pertinent information

13. Describe the purpose of EMS radio codes and give examples of local radio codes. p. 107

    Designed to communicate a large amount of information quickly and accurately

    Allows transmission of information in a format not readily understood by the public

14. List radio techniques that improve efficiency. pp. 107–108

    Listen before using a channel to ensure it is not in use

    Key the transmitter button for one second before speaking

    Speak close into the microphone or directly across it

    Speak clearly and slowly

    Do not convey emotion

    Keep the message brief

    Protect patient privacy

    Confirm reception of the message

    Repeat important information back to sender

    Write down important information

    Do not use slang, salutations, or profanity

    Obtain confirmation that your message was received and understood

Communication of Medical Information

15. List the important components of the patient medical report. pp. 110–111

    Unit designation, personnel, and level of certification

    Scene description

    Patient's name, age, sex, height, weight

    Patient's chief complaint/primary problem

    Associated signs and symptoms

    Brief history of current medical problem

    Pertinent past medical history

    Findings of physical exam—

        vital signs, level of consciousness, ECG, trauma score, Glasgow Coma Scale, etc.

    Treatment rendered, time rendered, and results of care

    Estimated time of arrival

    Name of private physician

16. Prepare and present a sample patient medical report on a simulated patient. *pp. 110–112*

Describe the importance of written medical protocols.

Provide standard care process for various medical problems and situations

Reduce communication time

Backup for radio communications failure

Name five uses of the written EMS form.

Record of the patient's initial condition

Legal record of prehospital care

Documentation of refusal of care

Information for billing, chart review, etc.

Defense against malpractice

Prepare an EMS form based on a simulated patient.

(See Special Projects)

CASE STUDY REVIEW

Reread the case study in Intermediate Emergency Care *and then read the discussion below.*

This case review highlights some important aspects of radio communications during an EMS response and shows the value that state-of-the-art communications have in emergency medical service.

CHAPTER 5 CASE STUDY

An accident along Interstate Highway 20 demonstrates the various elements of an EMS communications system and the valuable service such a system provides. A cellular phone brings the report of the accident through the universal entry number 911. Because Duane is in an unfamiliar area, dialing 911 saves both precious time and brings Duane in contact with a trained dispatcher who has access to all the public safety services.

The dispatcher asks predetermined questions to identify quickly the pertinent information she needs to summon the appropriate personnel and equipment to the right location and to determine medical dispatch priority. She activates a predesignated response, electronically alerting EMS, fire, police, and rescue services. The computer-aided dispatch (CAD) system also provides each responding service with printed dispatch information, thereby eliminating any confusion regarding street names and directions.

Finally, the dispatcher returns to the caller to advise him to stay off the highway. If this were a medical call or had occurred on a safer stretch of roadway, she would likely provide Duane with pre-arrival emergency medical care instructions.

Ambulance 15 arrives first at the scene. The senior EMT-Intermediate assumes the role of incident commander. She does a quick scene survey, advises incoming units of the situation, and directs them to a staging area. Due to the multiple-agency response, her most effective means of communication would be a hand-held portable radio, operating on the mutual aid frequency. As soon as a fire officer arrives, the senior EMT-Intermediate would relinquish scene command so she could focus on patient assessment and care.

The senior EMT-Intermediate uses the ambulance radio to contact the trauma center and alert them to the accident, the number of injured, the nature and severity of injuries, and the estimated time of arrival at the emergency department. She provides further information on the patients as she departs the scene en route to the trauma center. This communication is possible through the use of a system-wide repeater system. If the signal from the ambulance is too weak to reach the distant trauma center, the ambulance radio will activate a remote tower that will then retransmit the signal to the hospital base station.

Upon arrival at the emergency department, the EMT-Intermediate gives a verbal patient care report (PCR) to the trauma team. This report is followed by complete documentation of the call on the ambulance report form. This form includes such information as the mechanism of injury, chief complaint, results of the primary and secondary survey, serial vital signs, pertinent patient history, and care provided at the scene and en route to the hospital. It will become part of the patient's permanent record, a document for quality improvement, and a legal record of the findings and actions of the EMS personnel on this call.

CONTENT SELF-EVALUATION

MULTIPLE CHOICE

_____ **1.** The main transmitter of an EMS radio system is generally located close to the antenna and is called the
   A. remote console.
   B. repeater.
   C. base station.
   D. satellite receiver.
   E. encoder module.

_____ **2.** The normal range for the mobile transmitter, without a repeater, is about
   A. 5 miles.
   B. 10 to 15 miles.
   C. 25 miles.
   D. 50 to 100 miles.
   E. 125 miles.

_____ **3.** The device that receives a radio signal and retransmits the message at a higher power level is the
   A. portable radio.
   B. mobile radio.
   C. repeater.
   D. remote console.
   E. none of the above

_____ **4.** The device that activates a radio to receive and recognize messages containing a certain signal or tone is called a(n)
   A. remote receiver.
   B. satellite receiver.
   C. encoder.
   D. decoder.
   E. none of the above

_____ **5.** The type of radio transmission that is strictly "line of sight" and less subject to atmospheric interference is called amplitude modulation (AM).
   A. True
   B. False

_____ **6.** A system that automatically routes transmissions to the next available frequency is called
   A. band management.
   B. frequency assessment.
   C. trunking.
   D. frequency encoding.
   E. frequency modulation.

_____ **7.** One of the more important skills of an EMT-Intermediate is to gather essential patient information, organize it, and relay it to the medical control physician.
   A. True
   B. False

_____ **8.** All of the following are appropriate for good EMS communications except to
   A. speak close to the microphone.
   B. speak directly into or across the microphone.
   C. talk in a normal tone.
   D. speak without emotion.
   E. explain everything in detail.

_____ **9.** If the portable radio you are using does not transmit from your location, attempt to
   A. move to higher ground.
   B. touch the antenna to something metal while transmitting.
   C. move toward a window or away from structural steel.
   D. A and C.
   E. all of the above

10. Which of the following should be addressed by state or local protocols?
   A. care steps for all major medical emergencies
   B. patients who refuse care
   C. non-EMS physicians on the scene
   D. "Do Not Resuscitate" orders
   E. all of the above

11. The time needed to send an adequate ECG strip via telemetry is about
   A. 15 to 20 seconds.
   B. 20 to 30 seconds.
   C. 30 to 45 seconds.
   D. one minute.
   E. none of the above

12. The written run report may become
   A. a record of the patient's initial condition.
   B. a legal record of prehospital care.
   C. the source of essential information for billing, etc.
   D. documentation of a patient's refusal of care.
   E. all of the above

SEQUENCING

13. Place the following sequence of events in prehospital care in the order in which they would occur. Number the first event 1, the second event 2, and so on.

_____ A. treatment and preparation for transport

_____ B. preparation for the next event

_____ C. occurrence and detection

_____ D. notification and response

DESCRIPTION

14. List at least two responsibilities of the Federal Communications Commission.

_____

_____

15. List at least three responsibilities of the EMS dispatcher.

_____

_____

SPECIAL PROJECT

The authoring of both the radio message to the receiving hospital and the written run report are two of the most important tasks you will perform as an EMT-Intermediate. Read the following paragraphs, compose a radio message, and complete the run report for this call.

The Call:
At 3:15 P.M., your ambulance, Unit 89, is paged out to an unconscious person at the local baseball field on a very hot (97°), humid Saturday. You are accompanied by EMT-Intermediate Steve Phillips, your partner for the day.

You arrive on scene at 3:22 to find a young male collapsed at third base. You find him to be unconscious, perspiring heavily, and with skin cool to the touch. You remove a pillow under the boy's head, placed there by bystanders. The airway is clear, breathing adequate, and the pulse rapid and bounding. One bystander says, "He was playing ball and just collapsed." Another young bystander identifies himself as the victim's brother and states that "nothing like this has happened before." He identifies his brother as 13-year-old John Thompson. He lives about a mile away.

The rest of the assessment reveals no signs of trauma. Blood pressure is 136/98, pulse 92 and strong. The ECG traces normal sinus rhythm. Respirations are 24 and normal in depth and pattern (at 3:27). The young boy responds to painful stimuli, but not to verbal command or his name. You note pupils to be equal and slow to react. You apply oxygen at 4 liters by nasal cannula, and move the patient into the shade.

You contact the receiving hospital and call in the following report:

_____

_____

_____

_____

_____

_____

_____

_____

Expected ETA is 20 minutes.

Medical control at the receiving hospital orders you to start an IV line with normal saline at a TKO rate. You repeat the orders to medical control and then begin your care. Your first IV attempt on the right forearm is unsuccessful; the second attempt on the left forearm gets a flashback and infuses well. You retake vitals. The patient is now responding to verbal stimuli, the BP is 134/96, pulse 90, ECG reads NSR, respirations 24. The patient is loaded on the stretcher at 3:37 and moved to the ambulance.

You contact medical control and provide the following update:

_____

_____

_____

_____

_____

_____

_____

_____

ETA 10 minutes

En route vitals (3:45) are BP 132/90, ECG reads NSR, pulse 88, respirations at 24. The patient is now conscious and alert, although he cannot remember the incident. The trip is uneventful, and you arrive at the hospital at 3:57. You transfer the responsibility for the patient to the emergency physician. You then restock and wipe out the ambulance and report it back in service at 4:15. You now sit down to write the run report.

Complete the run report on the following page from the information contained in the narrative of this call.

(Compare the radio communication and run-report form that you prepared against the example in the answer key section of this workbook. As you make this comparison, keep in mind that there are many "correct" ways to communicate this body of information. Ensure that you have recorded the major points to describe the patient and his condition at all stages of the run.)

Date / /	Emergency Medical Services Run Report	Run # 911

Patient Information   **Service Information**   Times

Name:	Agency:	Rcvd :
Address:	Location:	Enrt :
City: St: Zip:	Call Origin:	Scne :
Age: Birth: / / Sex: [M][F]	Type: Emrg[ ] Non[ ] Trnsfr[ ]	LvSn :
Nature of Call:		ArHsp :
Chief Complaint:		InSv :

Description of Current Problem:

Medical Problems

Past		Present
[ ]	Cardiac	[ ]
[ ]	Stroke	[ ]
[ ]	Acute Abdomen	[ ]
[ ]	Diabetes	[ ]
[ ]	Psychiatric	[ ]
[ ]	Epilepsy	[ ]
[ ]	Drug/Alcohol	[ ]
[ ]	Poisoning	[ ]
[ ]	Allergy/Asthma	[ ]
[ ]	Syncope	[ ]
[ ]	Obstetrical	[ ]
[ ]	GYN	[ ]

Other:

Trauma Scr: Glascow:

On Scene Care:	First Aid:
	By Whom?

02 @ L : Via	C-Collar :	S-Immob. :	Stretcher :

Allergies/Meds:	Past Med Hx:

Time	Pulse	Resp.	BP S/D	LOC	ECG
:	R: [r][i]	R: [s][l]	/	[a][v][p][u]	
Care/Comments:					
:	R: [r][i]	R: [s][l]	/	[a][v][p][u]	
Care/Comments:					
:	R: [r][i]	R: [s][l]	/	[a][v][p][u]	
Care/Comments:					
:	R: [r][i]	R: [s][l]	/	[a][v][p][u]	
Care/Comments:					

Destination:	Personnel:	Certification
Reason:[ ]pt [ ]Closest [ ]M.D. [ ]Other	1.	[P][E][O]
Contacted: [ ]Radio [ ]Tele [ ]Direct	2.	[P][E][O]
Ar Status: [ ]Better [ ]UnC [ ]Worse	3.	[P][E][O]

CHAPTER 6

GENERAL PATIENT ASSESSMENT AND INITIAL MANAGEMENT

PART I (pages 115–137)

REVIEW OF CHAPTER 6 OBJECTIVES

After reading this chapter, you should be able to do the following:

A Systematic, Thorough Approach

1. **Understand the importance of a step-by-step approach to high-quality prehospital intermediate life support.** pp. 116–118

Assures a thorough and complete assessment that identifies all significant patient problems and symptoms

Enables an EMT-Intermediate to correct life-threatening situations and to establish the priorities of care

Assures continuity of care through communication to the emergency department

General Phases of Assessment

2. **Identify the information gathered in each phase of patient assessment.** pp. 118–119

Review of dispatch information

Location of the call

Nature of the call

Equipment that may be needed

Other units that may be responding

Scene survey/environmental safety

Hazards to personal and patient safety

Mechanism of injury

Number of patients

Additional resources needed

Primary assessment

Rapid identification of life-threatening injuries/problems

Rapid correction of life-threatening injuries/problems

Determination of the priority for transport

Secondary assessment

Head-to-toe evaluation for the signs of injury

Verbal questioning for symptoms

Inspection, palpation, auscultation, and percussion

Vital signs

Pulse rate and quality

Respiratory rate, depth, and effort

Blood pressure

Temperature—core and peripheral

Patient history

History of previous illness

Past medical history

Medications

Allergies

Personal physician

Review of Dispatch Information

3. Describe the type of information that can be obtained from a careful evaluation of the dispatcher's information. *pp. 119–120*

Type of run (medical vs. trauma)

Seriousness

Multiple patient incidents

Hazardous material incidents

Crime scenes

Patient age and sex

Chief complaint and significant history

Scene Survey/Environmental Safety

4. List some of the potential scene hazards that need to be ruled out to ensure safe patient care. *pp. 120–122*

Violent or armed patients

Traffic hazards

Electrical hazards

Fire hazards

Explosion hazards

Toxic chemicals (inhalation, contamination, or burns)

Adverse surface conditions (extreme heights or depths, debris, oil, etc.)

Adverse weather conditions

Structural collapse

Airborne or bloodborne pathogens

Primary Assessment

5. Describe the A, B, C, D, and E of the primary assessment. *pp. 123–135*

Airway and cervical spine control—Ensures that the trauma patient's spine is stabilized and that the airway is maintained and clear of obstruction (In the unconscious patient, this may involve patient positioning or include basic and advanced airway procedures such as oral airway or endotracheal tube placement.)

Breathing—Ensures that respirations are adequate in volume and rate (Breathing may be assisted with supplemental oxygen or provided by bag-valve-mask.)

Circulation—Determines if capillary refill is more than 3 seconds, if the skin is cool and clammy, if pulses are rapid and weak, or if distal pulses are absent (If such signs suggest shock, elevate the patient's legs and consider the use of PASG. Stop any obvious and severe hemorrhage.)

Disability—Determines the patient's level of consciousness (AVPU). Check for signs of neurologic deficit. (Ensure that the cervical spine is immobilized early in the assessment if there is any reason to suspect spine injury.)

Expose—Enables a quick look at the entire patient for any signs of potentially life-threatening injury, including hemorrhage or head, neck, chest, or abdominal injury

6. Identify the life-threatening conditions that can be identified and corrected during the primary assessment. *pp. 135–137*

Partial and complete airway obstruction

Flail chest

Open pneumothorax

Tension pneumothorax

Apnea, dyspnea, hypoxia

Hemorrhage

Hypovolemic shock

7. Identify conditions and injuries that require immediate and rapid hospital transport. *pp. 136–137*

Importance of the Golden Hour in cases of trauma

Use of Glasgow Coma Scale and Trauma Score to help set priorities for patient care

CASE STUDY REVIEW

Reread the case study in Intermediate Emergency Care *and then read the discussion below.*

This case study examines an assault and applies the elements of response that have been addressed within this chapter. Included in this case study are the dispatch information, scene survey, primary assessment, determination of the need for rapid transport or on-scene care, and some of the steps of immediate patient stabilization as called for by the primary survey.

CHAPTER 6 CASE STUDY

Pam and Mike listen carefully to the dispatch information as they prepare to respond. They note the "unfriendly" part of town and agree that they will not arrive at the scene until the police secure it. The nature of the call, "assault," tells them to expect trauma: a gunshot, knife wound, or blunt trauma from a fist fight. Pam accesses the trauma kit and reviews the regional trauma protocols while Mike drives to the scene.

There is excitement at the scene as the EMT-Intermediates arrive. However, the assessment process drilled into Pam and Mike during their training and few years of experience ensures that they will follow an organized and ordered step-by-step assessment process. They will employ the A, B, C, D, and E of the primary assessment and then determine the patient's need for immediate care and transport.

Pam assumes responsibility for the primary assessment, while Mike stabilizes the head and neck. Pam clears the airway with suction and inserts the oral airway. She then moves to the next primary assessment step: breathing. The patient is breathing with rapid, shallow breaths. Pam exposes the chest and discovers a sucking chest wound. She quickly seals the wound while Mike begins ventilation with a bag-valve-mask.

Pam notices that the patient's radial pulse is strong. This sign suggests the patient's circulatory status is stable for now. Through her experience, Pam knows that the body compensates well for blood loss, especially in younger patients. She continues to monitor both the vital signs and the patient's level of consciousness for any signs of deterioration.

Pam relays the findings of her primary assessment to paramedic Mark Rogers. She tells him of the sealed pneumothorax, the absence of breath sounds on the right side, the patient's circulatory status, and his level of consciousness. The patient's level of consciousness and the penetrating chest injury both require immediate transport to the trauma center.

MULTIPLE CHOICE

_____ **1.** A relatively complete patient assessment needs to be employed with both medical and trauma patients for many reasons, including
   A. trauma may be caused by a medical problem.
   B. an apparent medical problem may have a traumatic origin.
   C. medical problems may have significant physical signs.
   D. pre-existing medical problems increase the impact of trauma.
   E. all of the above

_____ **2.** The scene survey should include all of the following except
   A. identification of mechanism of injury.
   B. identification of hazards.
   C. assessment of the patient for life-threatening problems.
   D. locating all potential patients.
   E. determination of any additional assistance needed.

_____ **3.** The major goal of the primary assessment is to
   A. score the patient's condition.
   B. identify care delivered in the "Golden ten-minutes."
   C. determine whether trauma-center care is needed.
   D. correct life threats and determine the need for immediate transport.
   E. identify the signs and symptoms of shock.

_____ **4.** The first step of the primary assessment is
   A. airway assessment.
   B. breathing assessment.
   C. circulatory function assessment.
   D. airway assessment with cervical spine stabilization.
   E. cervical spine stabilization.

_____ **5.** All of the following are characteristics of normal respiration except
   A. volume of 500 mL.
   B. minimal abdominal movement.
   C. rate of 12 to 20/min.
   D. irregular pattern.
   E. quiet and unobtrusive.

_____ **6.** Which of the following pulses would be the last to be lost as a patient moves into shock?
   A. brachial
   B. radial
   C. carotid
   D. temporal
   E. tibial

_____ **7.** The "expose" of the primary assessment examines the patient to determine
   A. if significant external hemorrhage is occurring.
   B. if there is obvious deformity, edema, or discoloration.
   C. if there are any other life-threatening injuries.
   D. all of the above
   E. none of the above

_____ **8.** Which of the following conditions is not a reason to consider rapid transport?
   A. threat to respiratory function
   B. signs or symptoms of shock
   C. neurologic deficit
   D. uncorrectable airway problem
   E. respiratory rate of 18

SEQUENCING

9. Place the phases of patient assessment in proper order. Number the steps from 1–6.

_____ **A.** secondary assessment

_____ **B.** vital signs determination

_____ **C.** scene survey

_____ **D.** primary assessment

_____ **E.** dispatch information review

_____ **F.** patient history

10. Place the following in order of decreasing level of consciousness. Number the steps from 1 to 4.

_____ **A.** unresponsive

_____ **B.** responds to verbal stimuli

_____ **C.** responds to painful stimuli

_____ **D.** alert

DESCRIPTION

11. Identify information that can be gained from the dispatcher.

_____

_____

_____

_____

12. Identify information that the scene survey may provide.

_____

_____

_____

_____

SPECIAL PROJECT

The authoring of radio messages to medical control is one of the most important tasks that you will perform as an EMT-Intermediate. Read the following information. Then compose an initial and an updated radio message that you might send to medical control.

The Call:

At 6:32 P.M., dispatch pages medic rescue unit 21 and sends the unit to a one-car accident at the corner of Elm and Wildwood Lane. One patient is reported unconscious. The fire department is also en route.

You and your partner, Mike Grailing, arrive with the ambulance at 6:45 and find that there are wires down, fuel spilling from the gas tank, and window glass around the scene. Bystanders state that the car swerved wildly, then hit the power pole. You notice there are no skid marks. You await arrival of the fire department, which will secure the scene.

Once the scene is safe, you and your partner approach. The patient is sitting behind the driver's seat with his eyes closed. He is unrestrained. Your partner employs a jaw thrust with cervical precautions and cervical immobilization. You now begin the assessment. You notice a break in the car's windshield and a small contusion on your patient's forehead. He is unconscious, has a strong pulse, and displays minor respiratory wheezing and stridor. Assessment of the neck reveals a small welt but no other apparent injuries. The pupils are equal and reactive. Oxygen is administered at 12 L per minute via nonrebreather mask, and initial vitals (respiratory rate of 24 with audible wheezes, BP of 110/76, strong pulse of 90, and oxygen saturation of 94%) are taken at 6:52. The ECG displays normal sinus rhythm.

The patient awakens and asks, "What happened?" He thinks he was stung by a bee. Last year he had a similar reaction to a bee sting and has a kit at home that his physician prescribed for him. The patient complains of itching. You notice hives starting to form.

Based upon protocol, you initiate the IV run T.K.O. with lactated Ringer's solution in the right forearm using a 16-gauge over-the-catheter needle while the patient is being immobilized and moved to a long spineboard.

Medical control is contacted, and you call in the following:

_____

_____

_____

_____

_____

_____

_____

_____

_____

_____

_____

_____

Just prior to movement to the ambulance (6:59), the patient is monitored and found to have the following vitals: BP 118/88, pulse 78 strong and regular, respirations 20 and regular with clear breath sounds, an ECG showing a normal sinus rhythm, and a pulse oximetry reading of 99%.

The patient history, which is taken at the scene and during transport, reveals that the patient is William Sobeski. He is 28 years old and lives at 2145 East Brookline Drive in the city of Rochester. The patient denies any allergy except to bee stings. He was stung by a bee a year ago and was rushed to the emergency department because he "couldn't catch his breath." He denies any headache, visual disturbances, and any numbness and tingling. He also denies taking any prescribed medications other than that prescribed for bee stings. He has not eaten since noon. He requests Community Hospital because his sister works there.

Contact medical control and provide the following update:

_____
_____
_____
_____
_____
_____
_____
_____
_____
_____
_____

CHAPTER 6

GENERAL PATIENT ASSESSMENT AND INITIAL MANAGEMENT

PART II (pages 137–156)

REVIEW OF CHAPTER 6 OBJECTIVES

After reading this chapter, you should be able to do the following:

Secondary Assessment of the Trauma Patient

8. Describe the methods of conducting a prehospital physical examination. *pp. 137–139*

Inspection—observation of the patient's body for signs of injury or disease such as deformities, contusions, lacerations, discolorations, bleeding, etc.

Palpation—feeling of a patient's body for deformities, temperature variation, crepitation, masses, guarding, tenderness, etc.

Auscultation—listening through a stethoscope to breath sounds generated by the patient, such as rales, rhonchi, and wheezes

9. Identify the steps in conducting a head-to-toe physical examination. *pp. 139–155*

Head—examination of the ears, eyes, facial bones, nose, and mouth for signs of injury or medical problems, including:

Battle's sign

Bilateral periorbital ecchymosis (raccoon eyes)

Cerebrospinal fluid (CSF) drainage

Pupillary size, response, and tracking

Instability

Swelling, discoloration, hemorrhage, wounds

Neck—examination of the neck for the following:

Jugular vein distention

Tracheal deviation

Crepitation

Swelling, discoloration, hemorrhage, wounds

Chest and upper back—examination of the chest and upper back for the following:

Symmetry, bilateral excursion

Retraction, paradoxical movement, sucking chest wounds

Rales, rhonchi, wheezes, diminished or unequal breath sounds

Respiratory rate, depth, and pattern

Instability, crepitation

Swelling, discoloration, hemorrhage, wounds

Abdomen and lower back—examination of the abdomen and lower back for the following:

Symmetry, pulsation

Diaphragmatic breathing

Tenderness, rebound tenderness, guarding, or distention

Swelling, discoloration, hemorrhage, wounds

Evisceration

Pelvis—examination of the pelvis for the following:

Crepitation, instability

Swelling, discoloration, hemorrhage, wounds

Genitalia—examination of the genitalia for the following:

Swelling, discoloration, hemorrhage, wounds, discharge

Lower extremities—examination of the lower extremities for the following:

Distal pulse, capillary refill, neurologic deficit

Instability, crepitation

Swelling, discoloration, hemorrhage, wounds

Upper extremities—examination of the upper extremities for the following:

Distal pulse, capillary refill, neurologic deficit

Instability, crepitation

Swelling, discoloration, hemorrhage, wounds

10. **Discuss the evaluation of the four prehospital vital signs.** *pp. 155–159*

Blood pressure—suggests the effectiveness of the circulatory system (In adults, systolic blood pressure above 140 mmHg or diastolic above 90 mmHg suggest hypertension.)

Pulse—irregularities in rate and strength may suggest stress, shock, head injury, or other problems (A normal pulse rate is between 60 and 100 beats per minute. Children have a faster heart rate, while well-conditioned atheletes have slower rates.)

Respirations—rate, volume, and pattern used to determine the effectiveness and efficiency of respiratory effort (Normal respirations in the adult occur at 12 to 20 breaths per minute, with each breath moving about 500 mL of air. In the child, the rate is faster, while the volume of each breath is lower.)

Skin condition—provides indication of the body's ability to generate and dissipate heat to maintain a standard internal environment at 37°C (The skin should be pink, warm, and dry to the touch.)

Secondary Assessment of the Medical Patient

11. **Cite some of the differences in assessing the primary assessment for the medical and trauma patients.** *pp. 159–160*

Trauma patient—assessed through the primary survey to determine whether he or she would be best served by rapid transport or on-scene care; need to examine mechanism of injury, the signs or symptoms of serious internal or external injury, and the status of airway, breathing, and circulation

Medical patient—assessed to determine any immediate life threat—such as ectopic pregnancy—which may demand immediate transport; need to determine the problem affecting the patient through signs, symptoms, and patient history, since the mechanism of injury may not be apparent

12. **List the steps in conducting a patient history.** *p. 160*

Introductions

Chief complaint

History of present illness

Past medical history

Family and social history

13. **Identify the questions that should be asked for a pertinent patient history.** *pp. 160–163*

Chief complaint/history of present illness (PQRST)

Provocative and palliative factors: What events, actions, or circumstances might be related to the onset of pain or discomfort? What circumstances either increase or decrease the pain or discomfort of the chief complaint?

Quality of the chief complaint: How is the pain described by the patient? Is it gnawing, cramping, dull, sharp, etc.?

Region, radiation, and recurrence of symptoms: What is the exact location of the pain or discomfort? Is it moving or radiating?

Severity of symptoms: How severe is the pain as assessed by the patient's description and his or her reaction to it?

Time of symptoms: How long has the discomfort or pain affected the patient? Is it an acute problem or one that developed over time?

Medications

What prescribed medications is the patient using, what are they for, and could they be contributing to the current problem?

Past medical history

What pre-existing medical problems does the patient have? Are they pertinent to the current problem?

Allergies

What substances or medications is the patient allergic to, and could they be a contributing factor?

Personal physician

Who is the patient's physician, and what is the physician's specialty?

14. **Explain reasons for compiling a family/social history.** *pp. 161–163*

Identify heredity and lifestyle factors that may be related to or contributing to the patient's problem, such as smoking, substance abuse, or a family history of cardiac or hypertension disease

15. **Realize the importance of effective communication to quality patient care.** *pp. 163–165*

Prepare emergency department personnel for arrival of a patient and assure the continuity of care

Present information to support the appropriate care steps the medical control physician will order

16. **Explain how to prepare verbal and written patient reports according to the SOAP format.** *pp. 164–165*

Subjective information—information revealed by the patient, bystanders, and the scene

Objective information—information obtained through physical assessment of the patient

Assessment—statement of the EMT-Intermediate's general impression of the patient's condition

Plan—actions taken and proposal for managing for the patient

MULTIPLE CHOICE

_____ **13.** Battle's sign is reflective of what medical problem?
- **A.** periorbital ecchymosis
- **B.** basilar skull fracture
- **C.** cerebrospinal fluid leak
- **D.** cerebral concussion or contusion
- **E.** none of the above

_____ **14.** Pin-point pupils suggest which of the following medical problems?
- **A.** opiate overdose
- **B.** hypertension
- **C.** heat stroke
- **D.** A and C
- **E.** all of the above

_____ **15.** Distended jugular veins are suggestive of which of the following conditions?
- **A.** right-sided heart failure
- **B.** cor pulmonale
- **C.** tension pneumothorax
- **D.** pericardial tamponade
- **E.** all of the above

_____ **16.** _In caring for a patient with a traumatic chest injury, the trachea is found to deviate away from the injured side._ What problem would you suspect?
- **A.** flail chest
- **B.** tension pneumothorax
- **C.** airway obstruction
- **D.** cardiac tamponade
- **E.** all of the above

_____ **17.** _As you palpate a patient's chest you perceive a crackling sensation beneath the skin._ This finding would most likely lead you to suspect
- **A.** tension pneumothorax.
- **B.** pericardial tamponade.
- **C.** flail chest.
- **D.** tracheal deviation.
- **E.** paradoxical movement.

_____ **18.** The pain experienced by the patient when you release gentle pressure applied during palpitation of the abdomen is called
- **A.** Cullen's sign.
- **B.** Grey Turner's sign.
- **C.** rebound tenderness.
- **D.** guarding.
- **E.** referred pain

_____ **19.** Your assessment may reveal that a pelvic fracture exists when pressure is applied to the iliac crests. This fracture may present with
- **A.** pain.
- **B.** crepitation.
- **C.** instability.
- **D.** any of the above
- **E.** A and B

_____ **20.** If no distal pulse can be located, which of the following should be used to evaluate distal perfusion?
- **A.** skin temperature
- **B.** skin color
- **C.** capillary refill
- **D.** all of the above
- **E.** A and C

_____ **21.** The Glasgow Coma Scale will give the conscious and alert patient a maximum score of
- **A.** 12.
- **B.** 10.
- **C.** 15.
- **D.** 25.
- **E.** 100%.

_____ **22.** _A patient's pulse rate rises by more than 15 beats per minute when moved from a supine to a seated position._ This would indicate a blood loss of more than
- **A.** 100 mL.
- **B.** 250 mL.
- **C.** 500 mL.
- **D.** 1000 mL.
- **E.** 1250 mL.

_____ **23.** That which causes the patient (or someone else) to call for assistance is the chief complaint and is defined as his or her major
  A. discomfort.
  B. pain.
  C. dysfunction.
  D. all of the above
  E. none of the above

_____ **24.** The words crushing, oppressive, and gnawing are best categorized under
  A. intensity of the pain.
  B. quality of the pain.
  C. duration of the pain.
  D. location of the pain.
  E. quantity of the pain.

_____ **25.** The objective of radio communication between the EMT-Intermediate and medical control is the conveyance of just enough information to support the request for care and to allow the emergency department to prepare for the patient's arrival.
  A. True
  B. False

CHAPTER 7

AIRWAY MANAGEMENT AND VENTILATION

PART I (pages 169–193)

REVIEW OF CHAPTER 7 OBJECTIVES

After reading this chapter, you should be able to do the following:

Anatomy of the Respiratory System

1. Describe the anatomy of the upper airway, including: *pp. 172–175*

Mouth (oral cavity)—single cavity that serves as an auxiliary air passage; posterior upper surface includes the soft palate, which moves upward and closes off the passages from the nose to the pharynx during swallowing

Nose—hollow, two-sided chamber lined with mucous membranes; warms, filters, and humidifies air as it enters the respiratory system; openings include the nares, or nostrils

Pharynx (throat)—functions as the transitional area (passage) for food and air between the nose and mouth and between the esophagus and larynx

Epiglottis—flap-like structure covering the opening of the trachea (glottis); closes during swallowing to prevent food or fluids from entering the trachea and respiratory system

Larynx—tubular structure ("Adam's apple") that begins the lower airway; consists of the thyroid and cricoid cartilages, the vocal cords, the arytenoid folds, and the upper portion of the trachea

2. Name the three regions of the pharynx. *p. 174*

Nasopharynx

Oropharynx

Laryngopharynx (or hypopharynx)

3. Identify the relationship between the larynx and the tongue, pharynx, epiglottis, esophagus, and vocal cords. *pp. 174–175*

Tongue—found well above the larynx

Pharynx—airway chamber found directly above the larynx

Epiglottis—flap of tissue that covers the glottic opening of the larynx

Esophagus—found directly posterior to the larynx

Vocal cords—found within the larynx; form the glottic opening

Physiology of the Respiratory System

4. Discuss the following functions of the respiratory system. *pp. 178–180*

Mechanics of ventilation (exchange of gases between a living organism and its environment)

Lungs expand as the thoracic cage expands due to the contraction of the diaphragm, intercostal muscles, and other accessory muscles.

The elastic recoil of the lungs and gravity cause inspired air to be moved out of the lungs.

Pulmonary circulation

Right ventricle pumps blood depleted of its oxygen into the pulmonary artery.

Blood is directed to the respective lungs through the right and left pulmonary arteries, which then divide ultimately to the pulmonary capillaries.

Blood returns through the pulmonary veins to the left atrium.

Gas exchange in the lungs

Air brought into the lungs contains 21 percent oxygen and very little carbon dioxide.

Exhaled air contains about 14 percent oxygen and 5 percent carbon dioxide.

Diffusion of the respiratory gases

Oxygen in the inspired air diffuses across the alveolar space and then through the alveolar wall and the pulmonary capillary membrane where the oxygen attaches to the hemoglobin.

Carbon dioxide diffuses from the blood plasma in the reverse direction.

5. Describe oxygen transport in the blood, and cite factors that affect it. *pp. 180–181*

Oxygen is transported by hemoglobin found in the red blood cells. As it passes a well-oxygenated alveolus, 97 percent of the red blood cells are saturated. Very little oxygen is carried in or by the plasma of the blood. As the oxygenated blood passes the body's cells, the hemoglobin releases the oxygen.

Factors that affect oxygen saturation and transport include the following:

Inadequate alveolar ventilation—reduction of available oxygen at the alveolar level; may be caused by low oxygen levels in the air, respiratory muscle paralysis, chronic obstructive pulmonary disease (COPD), asthma, or pneumothorax

Decreased alveolar diffusion—caused by pulmonary edema, a condition in which fluid enters the space between the interior of the alveoli and the capillary; commonly increases the distance the oxygen must diffuse and hampers effective exchange

Ventilation/perfusion mismatch—results from lack of air exchange in some of the alveoli (as in atelectasis); unoxygenated blood from these alveoli mixes with the oxygenated blood from other areas of the lung. (*Note:* If the circulation is obstructed to some of the alveoli, such as in pulmonary embolism, a significant amount of blood is prevented from reaching the alveolar/capillary membrane.)

6. Discuss carbon dioxide transport in the blood and list factors that affect it. *pp. 181–182*

Approximately 66 percent of the carbon dioxide in the blood is transported as bicarbonate, 33 percent is transported attached to the hemoglobin, and about 1 percent is dissolved in the plasma.

Factors that affect carbon dioxide transport include the following:

Increased CO_2 production—produced by actions such as fever, muscle exertion, shivering, and metabolic acidosis

Decreased CO_2 elimination—caused by decreased alveolar ventilation from conditions such as drug induced respiratory depression, airway obstruction, COPD, and impairment of respiratory muscles

7. Describe the neurological control of respiration. *pp. 182–183*

Control of respiration by the involuntary nervous system through the use of stretch receptors in the tissue of the lungs and through chemoreceptors that monitor the oxygen and carbon dioxide levels in the blood and the pH of the cerebrospinal fluid

Increase in the stimulus to breathe from an increase in CO_2, a decrease in oxygen, or a decrease in pH

Decrease in stimulus to breathe from a stretching of the lung tissue (such as a deep breath)

8. **Describe the various measures of respiratory function and give the average normal values for each.** *pp. 184–185*

Tidal volume (V_T)—average volume of air inspired (or expired) with each breath, about 500 mL

Dead space volume (V_D)—portion of the tidal volume that does not reach the alveoli and is unavailable for gas exchange, about 150 mL

Alveolar volume (V_A)—amount of air that reaches the alveoli with each breath, about 350 mL

Minute volume (V_{min})—amount of air moved by the respiratory system with each breath (tidal volume) × respiratory rate

Functional reserve capacity (FRC)—maximum amount of air a person can move between a maximum inhalation and a maximum exhalation, about 4.5 liters

Respiratory Problems

9. **Describe the common causes of airway obstruction, and detail the special considerations of each.** *pp. 185–187*

Tongue—most common cause of airway obstruction; in the unconscious person, lack of muscle tone allows the tongue to rest against the posterior pharynx, and thereby obstructs the airway.

Foreign body—large, poorly chewed food and aspirated objects; most common cause of airway obstruction in children; often presents with the victim grasping his or her throat

Trauma—physical injury to structures of the upper airway; can be caused by objects such as teeth, tissue, or blood or by collapse of the airway due to penetrating trauma

Laryngeal spasm or edema—spasm of glottis (smallest portion of the airway) due to anaphylaxis, epiglottitis, and inhalation of toxic substances, superheated steam, or smoke; edema due to trauma

Aspiration—caused by aspirated vomitus, blood, teeth, etc.

Assessment of the Respiratory System

10. **Describe assessment of the airway and the respiratory system.** *pp. 187–193*

A continual, on-going assessment

During primary assessment, focus directed at detecting any potentially life-threatening airway problems. (*Note:* If the patient is not conscious, alert, and speaking, the airway and respiration are closely evaluated. The rate, depth, and symmetry of respiration are noted, as is the presence of any unusual respiratory sounds.)

During secondary assessment, focus directed at the finer details of respiratory evaluation, such as monitoring skin color, auscultation of breath sounds, checking for abnormal breathing sounds, palpation of the thorax, and using pulse oximetry and/or capnography

11. **Discuss pulse oximetry and end-tidal carbon dioxide detection, and describe the prehospital use of both.** *pp. 192–193*

Pulse oximetry—non-invasive monitoring of the arterial oxygenation of the skin; reflection of the oxygen delivery to the end organs provides oxygen saturation of the hemoglobin

End-tidal CO_2 detection (capnography)—accomplished either by a disposable device or an electronic sensor affixed to an endotracheal tube; measures the amount of CO_2 in the exhaled gas; disposable units change color while electronic detectors register a reading. (*Note:* In prehospital care, the presence of CO_2 reflects proper endotracheal tube placement. However, in patients without effective circulation the CO_2 levels may be very low.)

CASE STUDY REVIEW

Reread the case study in Intermediate Emergency Care *and then read the discussion below.*

The EMT-Intermediates in this case study deal with a patient in full cardiac arrest. While many aspects of intermediate emergency care are involved, the focus of this study is airway care and ventilation.

CHAPTER 7 CASE STUDY

Pete and Susan respond to a full cardiac arrest with a step-by-step team approach. They move deliberately through the ABCs of CPR and then progress into advanced life support procedures. Pete opens the airway and then determines that the patient is in respiratory arrest. Before moving on, he assures that an oral airway is inserted and that the patient is ventilated with 100 percent oxygen. He monitors chest rise and bag-valve-mask compliance to assure the patient is well oxygenated.

Susan determines that the patient is pulseless and immediately sets up the defibrillator. She delivers the first shock at 200 joules. Because of their quick actions, their patient responds with normal sinus rhythm (the normal heart rhythm) and, shortly thereafter, a carotid pulse.

When the patient does not begin respirations spontaneously, Susan suctions the upper airway and continues bag-valve-masking. Pete readies his equipment for intubation: the endotracheal tube, sized to the patient's little finger; the laryngoscope, with a #3 blade and brightly shining light; stylet to precurve the tube; tape to secure the tube; a 10-mL syringe to fill the tube cuff; and a stethoscope to auscultate for breath sounds once the tube has been placed.

Susan hyperventilates the patient for the few minutes preceding intubation, knowing that the 30 seconds without ventilation (while Pete places the tube) will cause some hypoxia. Pete quickly positions the patient's head, slides the laryngoscope into the right side of the patient's mouth, then slides it to the left, lifts the tongue, and visualizes the vocal folds. Susan applies the Sellick's maneuver, or gentle digital pressure downward on the cricoid cartilage. This pushes the opening of the trachea into Pete's line of sight and prevents aspiration. With his right hand, Pete passes the tube between the vocal cords and advances the tube about 1 inch past the cuff. He manually holds the tube in place while Susan attaches the bag-valve assembly and ventilates. He listens for and hears breath sounds on both the left and right sides. Susan stabilizes the tube, while Pete secures it with tape.

An end-tidal CO_2 detector is affixed to the end of the endotracheal tube. Its color change and the high oxygen saturation demonstrate that the tube is in the trachea. However, as the EMT-Intermediates move the patient, the tube displaces and becomes lodged in the right main stem bronchus. Susan pulls the tube back slightly, and bilateral breath sounds are heard and the oxygen saturation begins to rise.

Pete and Susan continue ventilations all the way to the hospital. They frequently evaluate the patient's pulse, breath sounds, the CO_2 detector color, and oxygen saturation while en route.

CONTENT SELF-EVALUATION

MULTIPLE CHOICE

_____ **1.** The nasal cavity is responsible for all of the functions listed below except
  A. warming the air.
  B. deoxygenating the air.
  C. humidifying the air.
  D. cleansing the air.
  E. the sense of smell.

_____ **2.** The space located between the tongue and the epiglottis is called the
  A. vallecula.
  B. cricoid.
  C. arytenoid fold.
  D. epiglottic fossa.
  E. glottic opening.

_____ **3.** Which of the following sequences correctly traces the passage of air during *inspiration*?
   A. trachea, larynx laryngopharynx, nasopharynx, nares
   B. nares, nasopharynx, trachea, laryngopharynx, larynx
   C. nares, nasopharynx, laryngopharynx, larynx, trachea
   D. laryngopharynx, nares, nasopharynx, larynx, trachea
   E. trachea, nares, laryngopharynx, larynx, nasopharynx

_____ **4.** The amount of air moved with one normal breath is called
   A. minute volume.
   B. alveolar air.
   C. tidal volume.
   D. dead air space.
   E. vital capacity.

_____ **5.** The oxygenated circulation that provides perfusion for the lung tissue itself flows through the
   A. pulmonary arteries.
   B. pulmonary veins.
   C. bronchial arteries.
   D. bronchial veins.
   E. none of the above

_____ **6.** The percentage of carbon dioxide in room air is approximately
   A. 10 percent.
   B. 4 percent.
   C. 0.4 percent.
   D. 0.04 percent.
   E. 0.10 percent.

_____ **7.** The majority of the carbon dioxide carried by the blood is
   A. carried by the hemoglobin.
   B. dissolved in the plasma.
   C. transported as calcium.
   D. found as free gas in the blood.
   E. bicarbonate, carried in the blood.

_____ **8.** All of the following conditions can cause reduced inspiratory volumes <u>except</u>
   A. pneumothorax.
   B. asthma.
   C. high-inspired oxygen concentration.
   D. respiratory muscle paralysis.
   E. emphysema.

_____ **9.** The normal oxygen saturation of hemoglobin in blood as it leaves the lungs is about
   A. 75 percent.
   B. 85 percent.
   C. 90 percent.
   D. 95 percent.
   E. 97 percent.

_____ **10.** The primary center controlling respiration is located in the
   A. medulla.
   B. pons.
   C. spinal cord.
   D. cerebrum.
   E. cerebellum.

_____ **11.** Which of the following would <u>not</u> increase the production of carbon dioxide?
   A. fever
   B. hyperventilation
   C. shivering
   D. metabolic acids
   E. exercise

_____ **12.** The reflex that responds to the stretch of the lungs by inhibiting respirations is the
   A. apneustic reflex.
   B. pneumotaxic reflex.
   C. Frank-Starling reflex.
   D. Hering-Breuer reflex.
   E. baroreceptor response.

_____ **13.** Which of the following is the <u>primary</u> stimulus that causes respiration to occur?
   A. increase in pH of the blood
   B. decrease in pH of the blood
   C. increase in pH of the cerebrospinal fluid
   D. decrease in pH of the cerebrospinal fluid
   E. reduced oxygen in the blood

_____ **14.** Which of the modified forms of respiration listed below is designed to expand the alveoli that may have collapsed during periods of inactivity or rest?

    A. cough

    B. sneeze

    C. hiccup

    D. grunting

    E. sighing

_____ **15.** Hypoxia may be caused by which of the following?

    A. smoke or toxic gases

    B. airway obstruction

    C. asthma, pneumonia, or emphysema

    D. shock or blood loss

    E. all of the above

LABEL THE DIAGRAM

16. Write the names of the components of the upper airway marked A, B, C, D, E, F, G, and H on the figure below.

A. _____

B. _____

C. _____

D. _____

E. _____

F. _____

G. _____

H. _____

Superior, middle and inferior nasal concha

NASOPHARYNX

Hard palate
Soft palate
A
B

OROPHARYNX

C

LARYNGOPHARYNX

D

E

F

H

Mandible

Hyiod bone

Thyroid cartilage

G

Thyroid gland

SPECIAL PROJECT

AIRWAY OBSTRUCTION

List the five causes of airway obstruction, and identify the mechanism that causes each problem.

1. _____

   _____

   _____

2. _____

   _____

   _____

3. _____

   _____

   _____

4. _____

   _____

   _____

5. _____

   _____

   _____

NORMAL RESPIRATORY VALUES

Identify the normal values for each of the items listed below.

	Inspired Air	*Alveolar Air*	
% Oxygen	_____	_____	PaO_2 _____
% Carbon dioxide	_____	_____	$PaCO_2$ _____

Normal Respiratory Rates/Volume:

Infant _____ to _____   Child _____ to _____   Adult _____ to _____

Tidal Volume _____

Alveolar Volume _____

Dead Space Volume _____

Minute Volume _____

CHAPTER 7

AIRWAY MANAGEMENT AND VENTILATION

PART II (pages 194–255)

REVIEW OF CHAPTER 7 OBJECTIVES

After reading this chapter, you should be able to do the following:

Basic Airway Management

12. Describe the procedures used to open the airway manually. *pp. 194–196*

Head-tilt/chin-lift (preferred technique in the non-trauma patient)—places one hand on the forehead gently tilting the head back, while the other hand is on the mandible, displacing it anteriorly

Jaw thrust (or the triple-airway maneuver)—places both hands on the lateral mandible, displacing it inferiorly and anteriorly (*Note:* If spinal injury is suspected, the head should not be tilted backwards.)

Jaw lift—places the rescuer's thumb into the mouth where the jaw and tongue are grasped between the thumb and fingers and are displaced anteriorly; requires care to ensure that the patient does not clench his or her teeth against the rescuer's thumb. (*Note:* Do not tilt the head with this maneuver if spinal injury is suspected.)

13. Discuss indications, contraindications, and methods for insertion and use of the following basic mechanical airways. *pp. 197–202*

Oropharyngeal airway—designed to maintain an airway by displacing the tongue anteriorly; should not be used for patients who are conscious or have an intact gag reflex; positioned by displacing the tongue forward with a tongue blade and inserting the oral airway along the base of the tongue (*Note:* The oral airway should be used when the patient is ventilated by any mechanical device.)

Nasopharyngeal airway—soft rubber tube that is lubricated and inserted posteriorly in the largest nostril; designed to be inserted into the nasopharynx in the unconscious or semiconscious patient; indicated in the semiconscious patient who requires airway management or in cases when an oral airway is indicated (*Note:* The oral airway should be used with care in the patient with possible skull fracture.)

Advanced Airway Management

14. Evaluate the advantages and disadvantages of the following *pp. 202–243*

Esophageal obturator airway (EOA)—blunt tube inserted into the esophagus; inflation of its large, soft, low-pressure cuff occludes the esophagus and prevents air from entering the stomach or stomach contents from exiting the esophagus; inserted blindly in a patient with the head and neck in the neutral or slightly flexed position (*Note:* The EOA should only be used in unconscious persons between $5 - 6\frac{1}{2}$ feet tall who do not have a history of esophageal disease, alcoholism, or caustic ingestion.)

Esophageal gastric tube airway (ETGA)—modified EOA, with an opening for the passage of a gastric tube; allows for gastric suctioning or relief of gastric distention secondary to positive pressure ventilation; indications and contraindications similar to the EOA

Endotracheal tube airway—single tube with one lumen passed through vocal cords; inflatable cuff at the device's distal end isolates the trachea from the larynx

Pharyngeo-tracheal lumen airway (PTL)—two-tube device, one tube of which isolates the oro- and nasopharynx while a second tube and cuff seals off either the trachea or esophagus; lumen of the tube allows ventilation if trachea is intubated (*Note:* While the PTL airway has many applications, it can be difficult to determine whether the distal tube is located in the esophagus or trachea.)

Esophageal tracheal combitube airway (ETC)—similar to the PTL airway, except that it is designed to be inserted into either the trachea or esophagus; occludes the passageway and the oral pharynx, isolating the trachea from the esophagus (*Note:* As with the PTL, EOA, and EGTA, the biggest drawback to this device is that the user must determine which tube the airway is in to assure the patient will be adequately ventilated.)

15. List the equipment used to perform endotracheal intubation. *pp. 207–208*

Laryngoscope handle and preselected blade

Magill forceps

Endotracheal tube in an appropriate size (and one larger and one smaller)

10 mL syringe

Stylet (if desired)

Bite block

Suction device

Tape or commercial tie-down

Bag-valve-mask

Stethoscope

CO_2 detector

Water soluable lubricant

16. Recall the indications, contraindications, and alternatives of endotracheal intubation. *pp. 213–215*

Indications—definitive method of choice for airway management; may also consider for patients with airway swelling related to an inhalation injury or trauma; may also be required for patients in need of assisted ventilation

Contraindications—an advanced skill that should only be attempted by someone with extensive training in the technique; contraindicated in the pediatric patient with epiglottitis

Alternatives—EOA, EGTA, naso- or oropharyngeal airway, PTL airway

17. Explain the need for rapid placement of the endotracheal tube. *p. 215*

A well-protected airway, such as with endotracheal intubation, is a very high priority in emergency medical care

The tube placement process denies the patient ventilation, hence the critical need to place the tube correctly and rapidly

18. Describe the methods used to assure correct placement of the endotracheal tube. *pp. 217–220*

Most definitive confirmation of tube placement—seeing the tube pass through the vocal cords

Immediately after tube placement—auscultation of both lung fields to assure bilateral breath sounds, auscultation of the epigastric area to ensure there are no gastric sounds, frequent repetition of auscultation during patient care

19. List and demonstrate the steps in performing endotracheal intubation. *pp. 215–220*

Assure the patient is being well ventilated by other means

Assemble equipment, including laryngoscope and blade, endotracheal tubes, tape, stylet, suction, BVM, 10 mL syringe, and Magill forceps

Test equipment, including laryngoscope light and tube cuff

Hyperventilate the patient

Insert the laryngoscope and visualize the vocal cords

Pass the endotracheal tube between the cords and advance it one-half to one inch beyond the distal cuff

Ventilate through the tube and auscultate both lung fields and the epigastrium

Inflate cuff with 5 to 10 mL of air

Tape the tube securely in place and note its depth in centimeters

Re-auscultate the lung fields and the epigastric area

Re-evaluate frequently for proper placement

20. State the precautions that should be observed when intubating a trauma patient. *pp. 228–230*

Suspect spinal injury

Provide all airway care with limited movement of the head and neck

Use a cervical collar

Hold the head in a neutral position manually while intubation is attempted

Consider oro- or nasotracheal intubation in such cases, as well as lighted stylet or digital techniques

Suctioning

21. Discuss the indications, contraindications, and methods of performing suctioning. *pp. 243–245*

Suctioning—use of pressures less than atmospheric to draw fluids and semifluids out of the airway

Indications—should be used any time it can effectively remove material from the airway

Contraindications—avoid continuous suctioning; draws against the patient's ventilation attempts and generally interrupts ventilation in the apneic patient

Methods—can be provided by electric or mechanical devices

Oxygenation

22. Discuss and describe the various oxygen administration devices used in prehospital care, and describe the advantages and disadvantages of each. *pp. 245–250*

Nasal cannula—provides oxygen concentrations between 24 and 44 percent at liter flow rates of 1 to 6 liters per minute; well tolerated by the patient, but administers only low concentrations of oxygen

Simple face mask—delivers oxygen at 40 to 60 percent concentrations with oxygen flow rates of 8 to 12 liters per minute; delivers moderate levels of oxygen, but muffles patient speech and may cause feelings of confinement

Nonrebreather mask—delivers 80 to 100 percent oxygen with flow rates of 10 to 15 liters per minute; delivers high concentrations of oxygen, but it muffles patient speech and may feel confining (preferred oxygen-delivery device for the hypoxic patient)

Venturi mask—delivers precise oxygen levels of 24, 28, 35, or 40 percent; ideal for the patient who needs a closely titrated oxygen flow

Ventilation

23. Discuss indications, contraindications, and methods for using the following devices: *pp. 250–253*

Pocket mask—provides some protection against direct contact with the patient and the patient's exhaled air; sealed to the patient's face with the rescuer's hands during ventilation

Bag-valve device—provides positive-pressure ventilation; sealed to the patient's face by one of the rescuer's hands, while the other hand squeezes the bag; best used for the intubated patient because the volume of air and the pressure delivered to the patient are low (*Note:* If the patient is not intubated, the air exchanged may not be enough to sustain life. Any time a BVM is used, it should have the oxygen reservoir attached and oxygen flowing at 12 to 15 liters per minute.)

Demand valve resuscitator—ventilates the patient with a flow of oxygen when a button or bar is pushed; can be used with face masks, EOA, EGTA, PTL airways, or endotracheal tubes; provides the patient with 100% oxygen (*Note:* The pressures at which it delivers oxygen may cause gastric insufflation or lung tissue damage. It is not recommended for patients who are intubated or the pediatric patient.)

Automatic ventilator—provides a patient with ventilation with 100% oxygen at a rate and volume determined by the user; recent advances in technology make automatic ventilators compact and dependable for field use (*Note:* These devices are not recommended for children under the age of 5 years and are dependent upon a good airway.)

CONTENT SELF-EVALUATION

MULTIPLE CHOICE

_____ **17.** In the head-tilt/chin-lift, the fingers under the chin should apply a firm pressure to ensure the jaw is displaced forward effectively.
   A. True
   B. False

_____ **18.** Which of the airway adjuncts act primarily by displacing the tongue forward?
   A. oropharyngeal airway   **D.** nasopharyngeal airway
   B. PTL airway   **E.** esophageal gastric tube airway
   C. endotracheal tube

_____ **19.** The EOA and EGTA have which of the following advantages?
   A. They are inserted blindly.
   B. They may be inserted without spinal extension.
   C. They are dependably inserted into the esophagus.
   D. They are inserted without other equipment.
   E. all of the above

_____ **20.** The cuff of the esophageal obturator or gastric tube airway is designed to occlude the esophagus and should be filled with a maximum of
   A. 5 mL of air.   **D.** 35 mL of air.
   B. 10 mL of air.   **E.** 50 mL of air.
   C. 15 mL of air.

_____ **21.** During the insertion of the EOA or EGTA, the patient's head and neck should be in the
   A. hyperflexed position.   **D.** extended position.
   B. flexed position.   **E.** B or C
   C. neutral position.

_____ **22.** The intent behind employing the Sellick's Maneuver is to
   A. displace the diaphragm.   **D.** clear an airway obstruction.
   B. increase venous return.   **E.** all of the above
   C. prevent regurgitation.

_____ **23.** The EOA or EGTA may be used with caution with all of the following respiratory arrest patients <u>except</u>
   A. persons under 16 years.   **D.** adult hypoglycemia patients.
   B. adult drug overdose patients.   **E.** adult patients with lowered mental status.
   C. adult hypovolemic patients.

_____ **24.** Which of the following are features of the PTL airway?
  A. It can be inserted blindly.
  B. It can seal off the nasal and oral cavities.
  C. Whether the tube is in the trachea or esophagus, the patient can be ventilated.
  D. It can be inserted without displacing the spine.
  E. all of the above

_____ **25.** Which of the following are benefits of the use of endotracheal intubation to secure the airway?
  A. Gastric distention is prevented.   **D.** Medications can be introduced.
  B. Complete airway control is achieved.   **E.** all of the above
  C. The trachea can be easily suctioned.

_____ **26.** The light of the laryngoscope should be a bright yellow and flicker slightly when pressure is placed on the blade.
  A. True
  B. False

_____ **27.** The tip of the curve of the MacIntosh laryngoscope blade is designed to fit into the
  A. nasopharynx.   **D.** arytenoid fossa.
  B. glottic opening.   **E.** epiglottis.
  C. vallecula.

_____ **28.** The major purpose for using a malleable stylet during endotracheal intubation is to
  A. maintain a pre-set curve in the tube.   **D.** prevent foreign matter from entering
  B. keep the tube's lumen open.   the tube.
  C. locate the esophageal opening.   **E.** all of the above

_____ **29.** When using the stylet for intubation, the tip of the device
  A. should extend 3 mm beyond the end of the endotracheal tube.
  B. should be even with the end of the endotracheal tube.
  C. should be recessed one-half inch from the distal tube end.
  D. is moved in or out during the intubation attempt as needed.
  E. none of the above

_____ **30.** To confirm the proper placement of the endotracheal tube, the EMT-Intermediate should
  A. watch the tube pass through the   **C.** auscultate the left lung field.
      glottic opening.   **D.** auscultate the right lung field.
  B. auscultate the epigastric area   **E.** all of the above
      during ventilation.

_____ **31.** Which of the following is <u>not</u> true regarding endotracheal intubation?
  A. The laryngoscope is held in the right hand.
  B. The laryngoscope is inserted in the right side of the mouth.
  C. The straight blade lifts the epiglottis.
  D. The curved blade fits into the vallecula.
  E. Advance the tube into the glottis, one half to one inch beyond the tube cuff.

_____ **32.** All of the following are common complicatons to the patient during endotracheal intubation <u>except</u>
  A. damage to teeth.   **D.** bronchial intubation.
  B. soft tissue damage to the   **E.** gastric distension.
      oropharynx.
  C. patient hypoxia during intubation attempts.

33. *Upon placing the endotracheal tube in a patient, you determine that you can only auscultate breath sounds on the right side.* You should
  A. withdraw the tube a few centimeters.
  B. withdraw the tube completely.
  C. pass the tube a few centimeters further.
  D. secure the tube and ventilate more aggressively.
  E. none of the above

34. *Upon placing the endotracheal tube, you hear very faint breath sounds and some gurgling over the epigastric region.* You should do which of the following?
  A. Advance the tube slightly.
  B. Withdraw the tube slightly.
  C. Inflate the cuff and auscultate again.
  D. Ventilate more forcibly.
  E. Place a second endotracheal tube.

35. Which of the following is <u>not</u> an advantage of nasotracheal intubation?
  A. It is well tolerated by a semiconscious patient.
  B. It is easier and quicker to perform than oral intubation.
  C. It can be placed without displacing the patient's head.
  D. The tube cannot be bitten.
  E. The tube can be easily anchored.

36. For which of the following patients is nasotracheal intubation contraindicated?
  A. patient with a potential spine injury
  B. patient not in arrest or deeply comatose
  C. patient with respiratory arrest
  D. severely obese patient
  E. patient with nasal fractures

37. In attempting digital intubation, the fingers of the rescuer must reach to the
  A. epiglottis.
  B. posterior nares.
  C. back of the tongue.
  D. laryngeal opening.
  E. cricoid cartilage

38. Which of the following is <u>not</u> required for blind nasotracheal intubation?
  A. a neutral or slightly extended neck
  B. a generally quiet environment
  C. a strong malleable stylet
  D. a patient who is breathing
  E. a preoxygenated patient

39. A danger to the rescuer associated with digital intubation is that the patient may bite down or clench his teeth during the process.
  A. True
  B. False

40. The use of a laryngoscope, and the passage of an endotracheal tube, may cause a child's heart rate to drop dramatically. This may reduce cardiac output and blood pressure.
  A. True
  B. False

41. In the intubation of children under 8 years old, it is recommended that the EMT-Intermediate use
  A. a cuffed endotracheal tube and a straight laryngoscope blade.
  B. an uncuffed endotracheal tube and a straight laryngoscope blade.
  C. a cuffed endotracheal tube and a curved laryngoscope blade.
  D. an uncuffed endotracheal tube and a curved laryngoscope blade.
  E. none of the above

42. Which of the devices listed below delivers the highest concentration of oxygen to the patient?
  A. nasal cannula
  B. simple face mask
  C. nonrebreather mask
  D. Venturi mask
  E. A and D

_____ **43.** Which of the devices below delivers the most controlled concentration of oxygen to a patient?
   A. nasal cannula
   B. simple face mask
   C. nonrebreather mask
   D. Venturi mask
   E. B and C

_____ **44.** The percentage of oxygen delivered to the patient when using the demand valve resuscitator is about
   A. 40 %.
   B. 50 %.
   C. 75 %.
   D. 90 %.
   E. 100 %.

_____ **45.** Hazards of using the demand valve to ventilate a patient include all of the following except
   A. oxygen toxicity.
   B. gastric distention.
   C. pressure-related injury.
   D. pneumothorax.
   E. subcutaneous emphysema.

_____ **46.** Which of the following is <u>not</u> an advantage of automatic ventilators?
   A. frees a rescuer when patient is not breathing
   B. convenience and ease of use
   C. dependability
   D. can be used on children below age 5
   E. light weight and tolerant to temperature extremes

SPECIAL PROJECT

PROBLEM SOLVING—AIRWAY MAINTENANCE

You have been called to a report of a man down and arrive with another EMT and one paramedic. You find bystanders doing CPR on a male in his mid-fifties in a parking lot. You take the patient's head and determine the bystanders are doing a fine job of ventilating the patient. You get out your airway bag and prepare to place an endotracheal tube.

What equipment would you prepare?

_____   _____

_____   _____

_____   _____

_____   _____

How would you check your equipment?

_____

_____

_____

_____

What would you ask the ventilator to do prior to your attempt?

_____

_____

Identify the steps of the procedure you are about to attempt.

1. _____
2. _____
3. _____
4. _____
5. _____
6. _____
7. _____
8. _____
9. _____
10. _____

You place the endotracheal tube. What actions would you take to ensure it is properly placed?

1. _____
   _____
   _____
   _____

2. _____
   _____
   _____
   _____

3. _____
   _____
   _____
   _____

4. _____
   _____
   _____

You place the endotracheal tube and notice no chest rise with the first breath. Auscultation reveals diminished breath sounds and gurgling over the epigastric area. What actions would you take?

_____
_____
_____
_____
_____
_____
_____
_____

CHAPTER 8

FLUIDS AND SHOCK

PART I (pages 256–276)

REVIEW OF CHAPTER 8 OBJECTIVES

After reading this chapter, you should be able to do the following:

Fluids and Electrolytes

1. **Identify the body's major fluid compartments and the proportion of total body water they contain.** p. 258–260

   Total body water (TBW)—accounts for 60 percent of the body weight, or about 42 liters in the 70 kg person; divided between two major compartments (intracellular and extracellular)

   Intracellular fluid (ICF)—accounts for 75 percent of body fluid

   Extracellular fluid (ECF)—accounts for 25 percent of body fluid; subdivided into two compartments (interstitial and intravascular)

   Interstitial fluid—accounts for about 17.5 percent of body fluid; remains outside the cells, yet not within the vascular space

   Intravascular fluid—accounts for 7.5 percent of body fluid; contained within the circulatory system

2. **List the major electrolytes, and discuss the role they play in maintaining fluid balance within the human body.** pp. 260–261

   Sodium—chief extracellular cation (positively charged particle); plays a role in regulating the distribution of water

   Potassium—chief intracellular cation; plays a major role in the transmission of electrical impulses

   Chloride—body's chief anion (negatively charged particle); plays an important role in kidney function and fluid balance

3. **Define diffusion, osmosis, active transport, and facilitated diffusion, and explain the roles they play in human fluid dynamics.** pp. 261–264

   Diffusion—tendency of molecules within a solution to move toward an equilibrium; keeps the fluids within each body compartment consistent in mixture

   Osmosis—movement of solvent (body water) from an area of lesser particle concentration to one of greater concentration; causes body water to follow the various electrolytes into the intracellular, intravascular, and interstitial spaces

   Active transport—biochemically powered movement of a substance across a cell's membrane, often against an osmotic gradient; essential activity of the cell membrane, which allows the body to control movement of electrolytes and essential molecules; faster than osmosis or diffusion, but it requires cell energy

   Facilitated diffusion—assisted transport across the cell membrane; mechanism by which glucose is brought into the body's cells

4. **Explain the ABO blood typing system and its significance to emergency medical care.** *pp. 265–266*

ABO blood typing system—identifies two antigens, which commonly occur on red blood cells; a person has one, both, or neither, and hence is classified as A, B, AB, or O (which is without) (*Note:* Since a person without an antigen of one type will have an antibody of that type and will react to blood with the antigen, typing is essential to ensure compatibility. An AB patient has both antigens and can accept any AB classification [universal recipient]. An O patient has neither antigen and can give blood to any ABO classification recipient [universal donor]. Because of the potential incompatibility of blood types, it is impractical to administer whole blood in the field.)

Abnormal States of Hydration

5. **Identify the abnormal states of hydration, and describe their common causes and effects on the human system.** *pp. 266–268*

Dehydration—net loss of body fluid may be caused by vomiting, diarrhea, disorders of absorption, fever states, diaphoresis, seeping wounds, or third space losses; can leave the cardiovascular system without the medium (plasma) to transport essential body materials effectively

Overhydration—net accumulation of fluid caused by the inability of the person to eliminate fluid (as in kidney failure) or an excessive intake of fluids (as in aggressive intravenous fluid administration); excess fluid flows out of the vascular space into the interstitial spaces and lungs causing peripheral edema or pulmonary edema

Fluid Replacement Therapy

6. **List the various fluid replacement products, and relate the advantages and disadvantages of using each one in the field.** *pp. 268–272*

Whole blood—ideal fluid replacement when blood is lost; precious commodity and carries with its administration the risk of reaction or disease transmission

Blood products—valuable in resuscitation of the patient who has lost fluid; carry the risk of reaction or transmission of disease

Colloids—solutions containing proteins or other large molecules that tend to remain in the vascular space for extended periods of time; draw water from the interstitial space and expand the vascular volume; tend to be expensive and have a relatively short shelf life

Crystalloids—solutions of electrolytes that have hypertonic (greater), isotonic (the same), or hypotonic (lesser) osmotic concentrations; remain in the vascular space for a relatively short time, but are inexpensive and practical to store; isotonic fluids most widely used in field because of limited side effects; commonly used isotonic fluids—lactated Ringer's solution, normal saline, and 5 percent dextrose in water

Acid-Base Balance

7. **Describe the acid-base balance system, and explain its impact on the human body as it applies during shock.** *pp. 272–274*

Systems that help mediate the pH of the human body—buffer system, respiratory system, and urinary system

Buffer system—chemically reduces the effect of adding or removing hydrogen ions

Respiratory system—removes or retains CO_2, which forms a weak acid when dissolved in water

Urinary system—retains or excretes bicarbonate, an alkali, to raise or lower the pH

Causes of failure of these systems:

Hypoventilation—may lead to respiratory acidosis

Hyperventilation—may produce respiratory alkalosis

Metabolic problems (such as failure of the circulatory system to deliver oxygen to the cells) or diarrhea, vomiting, or medications—may cause a metabolic acidosis

Medications or prolonged vomiting—may cause alkalosis (*Note:* A variation in pH of just 0.4 from the normal range of 7.35 to 7.45 may result in death.)

8. Name common acid-base disorders, and identify their causes. *pp. 274–276*

Respiratory alkalosis—caused by hyperventilation resulting from anxiety or head injury

Respiratory acidosis—caused by hypoventilation due to chest injury, head injury, or drug overdose

Metabolic acidosis—results from the accumulation of metabolic acids due to hypoxia at the cellular level; may be caused by hypoxia, hypoperfusion, diabetic ketoacidosis, poisonings, and serious infections

Metabolic alkalosis—results from an excess of bicarbonate ions; may be caused by ingestion of antacids or by prolonged vomiting and diarrhea

CASE STUDY REVIEW

Reread the case study in Intermediate Emergency Care *and then read the discussion below.*

This case study presents an example of aggressive and appropriate care for a patient who, by mechanism of injury alone, is suspected for the development of shock. It highlights the elements of both shock assessment and its care.

CHAPTER 8 CASE STUDY

Kent and Mary are called to a hunting incident involving a potential trauma patient in shock. Kent spends the time en route reviewing the local trauma protocols, and developing a plan of action for when he and Mary arrive. He also sets out and checks the equipment they will need if the patient is in shock. This will save precious time at the scene if the patient is seriously injured and needs immediate transport.

Kent and Mary find a young male named Jeff Hershey at the scene. Jeff is pale gray, anxious, restless, with a rapid weak pulse, slow capillary refill, and rapid shallow breathing. These are the classic signs and symptoms of shock and reflect the body's compensatory mechanisms that adjust for blood or fluid loss. These signs, along with the mechanism of injury, clearly establish a need for aggressive care and rapid transport to the closest trauma center. The EMS crew may very well be in a race against time to keep Jeff alive.

Kent and Mary both don sterile gloves and are very careful with their IV equipment. The amount of blood on the patient's jacket, blanket, and in the sheriff's car remind the care providers of the risk of bloodborne infection. Hepatitis, HIV, and several other diseases may be transmitted to Kent and Mary from Jeff's blood. Gloves should be worn with every patient, especially one with active hemorrhage. Ken and Mary should consider the use of eye protection or mask if blood splash is possible. Any needles should be promptly disposed of after use. Any contaminated material should also be disposed of properly or thoroughly cleaned. If a needle stick occurs or if there is direct contact with an open wound, the circumstances of the incident must be carefully documented and reported to the service infection control officer.

Kent begins the primary assessment. He ensures adequate breathing and applies oxygen via a nonrebreather mask at 15 liters per minute. This provides the patient with about 100 percent oxygen to increase oxygenation. Direct pressure is applied quickly to the site of hemorrhage. Kent will follow his manual bleeding control with a pressure dressing and will inspect the wound periodically to assure hemorrhage has arrested. As the primary assessment ends, Kent determines that the unit must move Jeff quickly to the trauma center.

In the ambulance, Kent and Mary raise Jeff's legs and cover him with a blanket. By raising the legs, they help to return blood to his central circulation and improve perfusion to vital organs. Blankets are necessary to help Jeff maintain body temperature. As the body compensates for blood loss, the normal thermo-regulatory functions of the skin are lost. The shock patient may become hypothermic very quickly.

En route, Kent inserts a large bore catheter into a large vein, connects it to a 1,000 mL bag of normal saline, and runs it wide open. If he were closer to the trauma center, Kent might consider a pressure infuser, but local protocol only allows 3 liters of prehospital fluid. Kent does however, get an order for a second IV line and third liter of fluid.

The care offered by Kent and Mary appears to be a very effective. They are able to move Jeff's blood pressure towards normal and deliver him to the Emergency Department with stable vital signs. He will probably tolerate his surgery well thanks to the swift and appropriate actions of Kent and Mary.

CONTENT SELF-EVALUATION

MULTIPLE CHOICE

_____ **1.** The intravascular fluid accounts for what percentage of the total body water?
   A. 7.5%
   B. 15%
   C. 35.6%
   D. 45%
   E. 75%

_____ **2.** Dehydration classically presents with all of the following signs <u>except</u>
   A. slow pulse rate.
   B. decreased blood pressure.
   C. excessive thirst.
   D. poor skin turgor.
   E. sunken anterior fontanelle (infants).

_____ **3.** The most prevalent extracellular cation is
   A. potassium.
   B. sodium.
   C. calcium.
   D. chloride.
   E. bicarbonate.

_____ **4.** The process by which a solvent travels through a semi-permeable membrane from a lesser concentration of solute particles to a greater concentration is called
   A. diffusion.
   B. active transport.
   C. osmosis.
   D. facilitated transport.
   E. facilitated diffusion.

_____ **5.** A solution that has an electrolyte concentration similar to plasma is called
   A. hypertonic.
   B. homeostatic.
   C. hypotonic.
   D. isotonic.
   E. none of the above

_____ **6.** The process that causes a solute to distribute itself equally throughout a solvent is called
   A. osmosis.
   B. diffusion.
   C. active transport.
   D. facilitated diffusion.
   E. permeation.

_____ **7.** The percentage of the blood that consists of red blood cells is referred to as
   A. its type.
   B. viscosity.
   C. the erythrocytic count.
   D. the hematocrit.
   E. none of the above

_____ **8.** The red blood cells account for what percentage of the formed cells of the blood?
   A. 62%
   B. 78%
   C. 86%
   D. 92%
   E. 99%

_____ **9.** If a patient has type A antigen and antibody B, he or she can generally be expected to safely receive which blood types?
   A. A and O
   B. B and O
   C. A and AB
   D. B and AB
   E. A only

_____ **10.** If a patient has type O blood, he or she can safely receive which blood types?
   A. A and O
   B. B and O
   C. AB and O
   D. A, B, AB, and O
   E. O only

_____ **11.** Which of the fluid replacement choices would be most desirable for the patient who is losing blood through internal bleeding?
- **A.** packed red blood cells
- **B.** fresh frozen plasma
- **C.** whole blood
- **D.** colloids
- **E.** crystalloids

_____ **12.** *A patient is in need of blood but there is no time to type and cross-match.* In this situation, the patient should be administered
- **A.** O negative blood.
- **B.** O positive blood.
- **C.** AB negative blood.
- **D.** AB positive blood.
- **E.** packed red blood cells.

_____ **13.** *You are transporting a patient who is receiving typed and cross-matched blood. The patient begins to display fever, tachycardia, and hypotension.* You should first
- **A.** warm the blood.
- **B.** administer epinephrine.
- **C.** slow the administration rate.
- **D.** mix the blood before continuing.
- **E.** stop the infusion.

_____ **14.** A solution for intravenous administration that contains proteins or other high-molecular-weight molecules is referred to as a(n)
- **A.** crystalloid.
- **B.** colloid.
- **C.** isotonic solution.
- **D.** hypotonic solution.
- **E.** hypertonic solution.

_____ **15.** Most of the solutions used in prehospital care for infusion are
- **A.** hypotonic colloids.
- **B.** isotonic colloids.
- **C.** hypertonic colloids.
- **D.** hypotonic crystalloids.
- **E.** isotonic crystalloids.

_____ **16.** Of the fluids listed below, which is <u>not</u> commonly used in prehospital care?
- **A.** 5% dextrose in water
- **B.** normal saline
- **C.** plasmanate
- **D.** lactated Ringer's solution
- **E.** A and C

_____ **17.** Increasing the pH value from 7.4 to 7.6 represents an increase in the strength of the acidity of a solution.
- **A.** True
- **B.** False

_____ **18.** The normal pH range for the human system is
- **A.** 7.00 to 7.50.
- **B.** 7.35 to 7.45.
- **C.** 6.90 to 7.65.
- **D.** 6.95 to 7.05.
- **E.** none of the above

_____ **19.** Which of the following systems is the first to respond to an increase in acidity and moderates the trend?
- **A.** the respiratory system
- **B.** the urinary system
- **C.** the buffer system
- **D.** the hepatic mediator system
- **E.** the circulatory system

_____ **20.** *A patient has been hypoventilating for quite some time.* The patient would be expected to have
- **A.** metabolic acidosis.
- **B.** metabolic alkalosis.
- **C.** respiratory alkalosis.
- **D.** respiratory acidosis.
- **E.** none of the above

SPECIAL PROJECT

Use the diagram to calculate and fill in the percentages of total <u>body weight</u> due to water for the fluid compartments marked A, B, C, D in the figure. Remember: the percentage of total body water for each compartment is as follows:

Intracellular fluid volume   75%
Extracellular fluid volume   25%
Interstitial fluid volume   17.5%
Intravascular fluid volume 7.5%

A. _____

B. _____

C. _____

D. _____

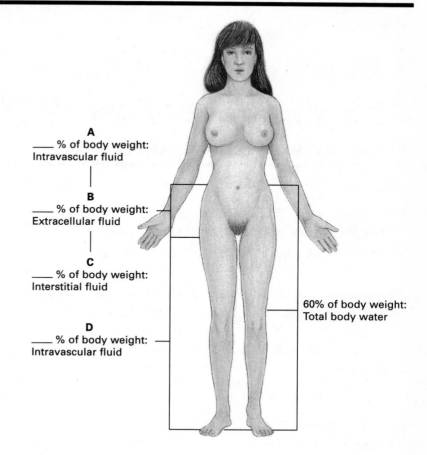

A
____ % of body weight:
Intravascular fluid

B
____ % of body weight:
Extracellular fluid

C
____ % of body weight:
Interstitial fluid

D
____ % of body weight:
Intravascular fluid

60% of body weight:
Total body water

CHAPTER 8

FLUIDS AND SHOCK

PART II (pages 276–309)

REVIEW OF CHAPTER 8 OBJECTIVES

After reading this chapter, you should be able to do the following:

Pathophysiology of Shock

9. Define shock from a medical standpoint. *p. 276*

Shock—inadequate tissue perfusion; inability of the human system, through the cardiovascular system, to supply the body's cellular needs

10. Describe the structure and function of the cardiovascular system. *pp. 276–280*

Structure and function—system of interconnected tubes, which direct blood to the essential organs and tissues of the body; powered by the central pump (the heart)

Importance—failure of any part places the body at risk

Causes of failure—when the tubes relax and can no longer direct the flow; when the fluid is lost to hemorrhage or plasma loss; when the fluid is no longer effective in its delivery of vital material, such as oxygen; when the pump fails to provide the power to move blood to essential tissues

Recognizing Shock

11. Explain the shock process, and describe some of the body's various compensatory mechanisms. *pp. 281–282*

Shock—results from many causes, but ultimately ends in inadequate tissue perfusion

Compensatory mechanisms for reduced fluid return to the heart, low fluid volume, and reduced cardiac output:

> **Increased peripheral resistance**—caused by constriction of blood vessels; provides two mechanisms to combat shock; first, constriction of the arterioles maintains blood pressure; second, it diverts blood to critical organs

> **Increased preload**—occurs when the veins constrict and reduce their volume; because veins account for about 60 percent of the blood volume, a reasonably effective response may result in modest to moderate blood loss

> **Increased heart rate**—response to lowering blood pressure; in the presence of low preload, may not be effective

> **Peripheral vascular shunting**—directs the blood away from the skin, conserves body heat, and reduces fluid loss through evaporation; also redirects blood to more critical areas

> **Fluid shifts**—result of drawing fluid from the interstitial and cellular spaces into the vascular space; although a slow process, can provide the vascular system with several liters of fluid

12. Identify the three distinct stages of shock. *pp. 283–284*

Compensated shock—initial response of the body to fluid loss; blood vessels constrict, the heart rate and strength of contraction increase, and blood is directed from less critical structures, such as the skin, to the internal and vital organs (*Note:* If the loss is not controlled, compensated shock will progress into decompensated shock.)

Decompensated shock—state in which the cardiovascular system is not receiving enough oxygenated circulation to maintain a compensatory state; blood vessels relax, the heart can no longer forcibly contract, and blood pressure and circulatory flow drop precipitously (*Note:* If immediate aggressive intervention does not occur, the patient will move into irreversible shock.)

Irreversible shock—state in which cell death has begun and the cardiovascular system is no longer capable of sustaining life; even if the lost fluid is replaced in its entirety (or the primary problem is corrected), damage is irreversible

Assessment of the Shock Patient

13. Describe and demonstrate the assessment of the shock patient. *pp. 285–290*

Look for the indications of shock

Observe respirations for rate and depth; note rapid, shallow breathing suggestive of shock

Carefully and deliberately assess pulse; suspect shock if pulse is rapid and weak, or if distal pulses are absent

Observe skin color, temperature, and capillary refill times (in children); note reduced peripheral perfusion, an early sign of shock

Assess the level of consciousness; reduced faculties, confusion, disorientation, or agitation should raise the index of suspicion for shock

Scan the body cavity, pelvis, and extremities for signs of injury that might contribute to shock

Prepare patient for rapid transport if the primary survey suggests shock

Maintain a constant and continuous vigil to recognize the early signs of shock

14. Name pertinent vital sign readings that indicate a potential shock patient. *pp. 291–293*

Blood pressure—falls late in the shock process, too late to be a useful indicator

Pulse—rises quickly as the patient loses blood and the body begins to compensate; pulse rate above 100, especially if it is weak, indicative of early shock

Rate of respirations—increases while depth decreases

Skin temperature—cool and clammy may reflect shunting of blood to the core circulation

Capillary refill time—greater than two seconds suggestive of shock

Management of Shock

15. Explain the indications for, and the initiation of, intravenous therapy. *pp. 296–299*

Indications—include the need for administration of intravenous medications, replacement of fluid loss, and obtaining venous blood samples for analysis

Initiation—begins with identification of an appropriate site, followed by the application of a venous tourniquet and the cleansing of the site for cannulation (*Note:* Steps then follow in this order. A catheter is selected, tape is torn to secure the catheter, and an IV solution and administration set are connected and prepared. The skin is pierced, the vein is entered [as denoted by flashback], and the catheter is advanced. The needle is withdrawn and the administration set is connected.)

16. List the equipment commonly used for intravenous therapy, and explain the purpose and use of each item. *pp. 299–304*

Venous tourniquet—used to obstruct the venous return, thereby dilating the vein and making cannulation easier

Cleansing agents (such as alcohol or Betadine)—used to cleanse the site, reducing the chance that infectious agents will enter the skin and blood vessel with cannulation

Catheters—most commonly over-the-needle variety, ranging from 24- to 14-gauge (smallest to largest); needle and catheter inserted into the skin and vessel, catheter threaded into the vein, and needle is withdrawn

Tape—torn prior to cannulation and used to secure the catheter, the connection between the catheter and the administration set, and the first few inches of administration set tubing

Administration set—tubing that carries the fluid from the solution bag to the catheter; contains a drip chamber and control valve that allow for controlling the rate of fluid administration; sets normally come in 60 (mini) and 10 (macro) drops per milliliter versions

Intravenous fluid—used to replace fluid a patient has lost and/or provide a carrier for drug administration; most common fluids for field use are lactated Ringer's solution, normal saline, and dextrose 5 percent in water

17. Identify the common complications of intravenous therapy, and describe the process of preventing or correcting those complications. *pp. 304–305*

Infiltration—due to extravasation of fluid; ensure that the catheter is within the vein and running properly

Hematoma—internal hemorrhage due to needle movement damage or delicate veins; withdraw the catheter and apply direct pressure

Pyrogenic reaction—reaction of agents within the solution with the patient's blood; results in fever, nausea, vomiting, chills, and backache; if suspected, discontinue IV immediately and save the solution.

Catheter shear—may occur when a catheter is drawn back over a needle that has been inserted into the vein; never withdraw the catheter over the needle

Air embolism—occurs when air is allowed to enter the vein through the administration set and catheter; completely clear the administration set of air and ensure that your IV solution does not run out

18. Identify the indications, contraindications, and application process for the PASG. *pp. 305–306*

Indications—indicated for any patient who displays internal or external hemorrhage in the lower abdomen, pelvis, or lower extremities; recommended for the stabilization of any pelvic and/or femur fractures or for the signs and symptoms of shock

Contraindications—should not be used in the patient who is experiencing pulmonary edema or who has a head or penetrating chest injury; use with caution on any patient who is experiencing dyspnea due to the pressure it may place against the diaphragm; do not employ the abdominal section if the patient is in the third trimester of pregnancy, has an abdominal evisceration, or has an impaled object in the abdomen

Application—assess breath sounds and record the patient's blood pressure, pulse rate and strength, and level of consciousness; visualize the abdomen, lower back, and lower extremities to ensure against sharp debris that could harm either the patient or the garment; apply the garment with consideration of the patient's injuries and position; inflate lower extremity chambers prior to or simultaneously with the abdominal chamber; follow local protocols for indications and contraindications

Communication and Transport

19. Understand the need for rapid transport of a shock patient, and name steps taken if on the scene more than 10 minutes. *pp. 306–308*

Need for rapid transport—should be executed within 10 minutes of the arrival of emergency medical services at the scene; weight of research in favor of improved patient outcome through quick delivery to a trauma center

Steps taken when on the scene more than 10 minutes:

Contact medical control and provide them with the mechanism of injury, patient vital signs, and the results of your primary assessment

Initiate IVs and begin to infuse fluids

Consider drawing blood for transport to the emergency department for typing and crossmatching

MULTIPLE CHOICE

_____ **21.** Which of the following can cause shock?
   A. heart attack
   B. infection
   C. spinal cord injury
   D. allergic reaction
   E. all of the above

_____ **22.** Adequate perfusion is dependent upon which of the following elements?
   A. the pump (heart)
   B. the volume (blood)
   C. the container (blood vessels)
   D. all of the above
   E. B and C

_____ **23.** The principle that accounts for a greater force of cardiac contraction when the heart is forcefully filled with blood and the myocardium is stretched is called the
   A. cardiac contractile force.
   B. Frank-Starling mechanism.
   C. Hering-Breuer reflex.
   D. rubber band syndrome.
   E. Boyle's law.

_____ **24.** Under normal conditions, the blood passing the alveoli will be oxygenated to what percentage?
   A. 65 to 70
   B. 75 to 85
   C. 90 to 95
   D. 97 to 100
   E. less than 65

_____ **25.** Which list places the stages of shock in the correct order of their occurrence.
   A. irreversible, decompensated, compensated.
   B. compensated, decompensated, irreversible.
   C. compensated, irreversible, decompensated.
   D. decompensated, irreversible, compensated.
   E. decompensated, compensated, irreversible.

_____ **26.** The major intent behind the mechanisms that compensate for shock is to
   A. reduce blood loss.
   B. reduce the vascular space.
   C. conserve oxygen.
   D. restore tissue perfusion.
   E. all of the above

_____ **27.** All of the following can cause hypovolemic shock except
   A. bowel obstruction.
   B. pancreatitis.
   C. cardiac dysrhythmias.
   D. ascites.
   E. peritonitis.

_____ **28.** The color, temperature, and general appearance of the skin can indicate shock before there are changes in the blood pressure.
   A. True
   B. False

_____ **29.** Normally capillary refill will occur within
   A. one second.
   B. two seconds.
   C. three seconds.
   D. four seconds.
   E. thirty seconds.

_____ **30.** The reduction in tissue perfusion that accompanies shock may cause hypoperfusion of the brain and in turn may cause which of the following?
   A. unequal pupils
   B. fever
   C. abnormal sensing
   D. disorientation
   E. all of the above

_____ **31.** The preferred position for the shock patient is
    A. supine with head elevated slightly.
    B. on the left side (left lateral recumbent).
    C. supine with legs elevated 10 to 12 inches.
    D. supine.
    E. on the right side.

_____ **32.** The volume of fluid infused using the macrodrip administration set is usually
    A. 5 drops per milliliter.
    B. 10 drops per milliliter.
    C. 25 drops per milliliter.
    D. 40 drops per milliliter.
    E. 60 drops per milliliter.

_____ **33.** *You have inserted an intravenous catheter, achieved flashback, and the IV does not flow.* Which of the following might be the cause?
    A. The catheter opening is up against a valve.
    B. The IV bag may not be high enough.
    C. The venous tourniquet has not been removed.
    D. There is an administration set valve closed.
    E. all of the above

_____ **34.** If the drip chamber is completely filled with fluid, the EMT-Intermediate should
    A. invert the bag and chamber and squeeze the chamber.
    B. apply pressure to the bag and let the fluid flow.
    C. run fluid through the chamber; the problem will self correct.
    D. discontinue the IV and start again.
    E. replace the administration set.

_____ **35.** *A patient you are attending, who has an IV in place and running, experiences fever, chills, nausea, and backache.* The patient is probably experiencing
    A. catheter shear.
    B. pulmonary emboli.
    C. an overhydration reaction.
    D. a pyrogenic reaction.
    E. none of the above

_____ **36.** Which of the following actions is likely to cause catheter shear?
    A. excessive movement of the catheter once in place
    B. withdrawing the catheter back over the needle
    C. using too large a catheter for the vein
    D. running fluid too fast
    E. contaminants in the solution

ANALYZING SIGNS OF SHOCK

Explain why these classic signs of shock occur.

Cool & clammy skin _____

_____

_____

_____

Agitation _____

_____

_____

_____

Rapid pulse _____

_____

_____

_____

Dropping blood pressure _____

_____

_____

_____

Ashen or cyanotic skin _____

_____

_____

_____

ANALYZING DROPS IN BLOOD PRESSURE

Explain why the blood pressure drops late during shock.

_____

_____

_____

_____

_____

_____

_____

APPENDIX I

DEFIBRILLATION

APPENDIX I OBJECTIVES

With each appendix of this workbook, we will identify the objectives and the important elements they describe. Review these objectives and refer to the pages listed if any points are unclear.

After reading this appendix, you should be able to do the following:

1. Describe the pertinent anatomy and physiology of the heart. *pp. 312–319*

Anatomy

Basic structure and location—four-chambered, fist-sized organ located in the center of the chest; two-thirds of its mass is to the left of the midline

Tissue layers—three tissue layers include the pericardium (the outer two-layered sac in which the heart sits), the myocardium (the heart muscle tissue), the endocardium (the heart's inner-most lining)

Chambers—four chambers include the right and left atria (which receive blood from the vena cavae and the pulmonary vein, respectively) and the right and left ventricles (which receive blood from their respective atria); ventricles form the major pumping chambers of the heart

Valves—two sets of valve pairs include the atrioventricular valves (which separate the atria from the ventricles) and the semilunar valves (which are between the ventricles and arteries into which they empty)

Great vessels—superior and inferior vena cavae meet at the right atrium and return blood from the upper and lower body, respectively; aorta receives blood pumped by left ventricle and distributes it to the major arteries of the body

Coronary circulation—distributes oxygenated blood to the myocardium through a series of small but very important coronary blood vessels; coronary veins drain deoxygenated blood into the left ventricle

Physiology

Cardiac cycle—left and right side of the heart work in unison; atria contract first, then, the ventricles; the relaxation or filling phase (diastole) begins the cycle, followed by the contraction phase (systole)

Cardiac output—volume of each cardiac contraction (stroke volume) times the number of cardiac contractions (heart rate) equals the cardiac output; blood pressure equals the cardiac output times the peripheral vascular resistance

2. Identify and explain the major elements of cardiac patient assessment. *pp. 319–323*

Common chief complaints and history

Common complaints—chest pain or discomfort, shoulder, neck, or jaw pain, dyspnea, syncope, or palpitations

Steps in evaluating pain—determine if the onset is sudden or gradual, identify its exact location (usually substernal), any radiation of the pain, the duration of the pain, the precipitating activity or circumstance, the type and quality of pain, any associated symptoms, any aggravating or alleviating factors, and any previous episodes of similar pain

Steps in evaluating dyspnea, syncope, or palpitation—determine the duration, onset, aggravating or alleviating factors, previous episodes, any associated symptoms, and any prior occurrence of a similar nature

Steps in eliciting a medical history—determine if the patient is taking any prescription medications regularly, is under treatment for any serious illness, has any heart condition, diabetes, hypertension, chronic lung disease, or allergies

Physical examination

<u>Look</u> for any sign of altered skin color or slow capillary refill, jugular vein distension, peripheral or presacral edema, or other indicators of prior heart problems

<u>Listen</u> carefully to breath sounds for rales, rhonchi, or wheezes

<u>Feel</u> the skin for diaphoresis and the pulse for strength, rate, and regularity

3. List at least eight causes of a poor ECG signal or tracing. *p. 331*

Excessive hair

Loose or dislodged electrode

Dried conductive gel

Poor lead placement

Diaphoresis

Patient movement or muscle tremors

Broken patient cable

Broken lead wire

Weak battery

Faulty grounding

Faulty monitor

4. Recognize the three cardiac arrest dysrhythmias that may call for defibrillation. *pp. 335–337*

Ventricular tachycardia—a rapid rhythm originating from a site in the ventricles

Ventricular fibrillation—a chaotic, unorganized rhythm originating in the ventricles; myocardium quivers and does not pump any blood

Asystole—absence of all electrical activity of the heart and, in turn, all muscular and pumping activity. (*Note:* In some cases, very fine ventricular fibrillation may appear as asystole. Confirm in at least two monitoring leads.)

5. List and explain the steps taken to manage the patient in cardiac arrest. *pp.338–347*

Initiate basic life support

Basic life support is the mainstay of resuscitation of the patient in cardiac arrest. Begin it yourself, or delegate it to someone else and monitor his or her performance.

Monitor the ECG rhythm

Evaluate the patient's ECG via quick-look paddles or monitor/defibrillation pads. Assure proper lead placement and good electrical contact. Evaluate the rhythm and obtain a tracing if possible. In an automatic defibrillator, the machine will automatically analyze the dysrhythmia to determine the appropriateness of shock delivery.

If indicated, defibrillate

If the patient's ECG displays ventricular fibrillation or ventricular tachycardia and no respirations or pulse, defibrillation is indicated. Assure that personnel are clear of the patient and possible electrical shock, and then deliver the defibrillation.

CONTENT SELF-EVALUATION

MULTIPLE CHOICE

_____ **1.** The skill of defibrillation once required advanced training. As such it was limited to use by physicians and paramedics. However, today it is performed by basic life support providers using automated devices.
   A. True
   B. False

_____ **2.** Which of the heart's chambers has the greatest mass of cardiac muscle?
   A. right atrium
   B. left atrium
   C. right ventricle
   D. left ventricle
   E. They have equal mass.

_____ **3.** The stroke volume is
   A. a measure of peripheral vascular resistance.
   B. the volume of a heart beat.
   C. the cardiac output divided by 60.
   D. the heart rate times cardiac output.
   E. the systolic quotient of myocardia activity.

_____ **4.** The pain most often associated with cardiac disease is located in the
   A. chest.
   B. jaw.
   C. back.
   D. flank.
   E. none of the above

_____ **5.** Which of the following medications would suggest a cardiac condition?
   A. nitroglycerin
   B. Maxzide
   C. Inderal
   D. Lanoxin
   E. all of the above

_____ **6.** Jugular vein distension should not be present when the patient is lying in the supine position.
   A. True
   B. False

_____ **7.** The intrinsic rate of the AV node of the heart is
   A. 100 to 180 beats per minute.
   B. 60 to 100 beats per minute.
   C. 40 to 60 beats per minute.
   D. 20 to 40 beats per minute.
   E. none of the above

_____ **8.** The ECG is an important tool in the evaluation of the patient with cardiac disease primarily because it indicates the relative pumping ability of the heart.
   A. True
   B. False

_____ **9.** Which of the following dysrhythmias is best described as a chaotic electrical activity with no cardiac pumping of blood?
   A. ventricular tachycardia
   B. ventricular fibrillation
   C. electromechanical dissociation
   D. asystole
   E. Smith-Parkinson-White syndrome

_____ **10.** Asystole is the absence of electrical activity and pumping activity. It presents with a flat line on the ECG and carries a dismal prognosis for resuscitation.
   A. True
   B. False

_____ **11.** Which of the following may cause cardiac arrest?
   A. drowning
   B. electrocution
   C. drug intoxication
   D. hypothermia
   E. all of the above

_____ **12.** An important factor influencing the success of defibrillation is
   A. the duration of ventricular fibrillation.
   B. previous counter shocks.
   C. paddle size.
   D. paddle placement.
   E. all of the above

_____ **13.** The initial electrical defibrillation should be set at
   A. 50 joules.
   B. 100 joules.
   C. 200 joules.
   D. 300 joules.
   E. 360 joules.

APPENDIX II

BLOOD GLUCOSE DETERMINATION

APPENDIX II OBJECTIVES

After reading this appendix, you should be able to do the following:

1. Identify the patients who are candidates for blood glucose determination. *p. 348*

Displays an altered mental status (*Note:* While low blood glucose states are commonly associated with diabetes, they may occur in other conditions as well.)

2. List the steps in determining blood glucose levels in the field. *pp. 349–353*

Follow universal precautions (don gloves)

Prepare the triggered fingerstick device

Locate an appropriate fingerstick site

Cleanse the site with alcohol and allow time for complete evaporation

Turn on the blood glucose determination device (glucometer)

Remove test strip from container and check expiration date

Lance the patient's finger and obtain a drop of blood

Touch a blood drop to the target area of test strip

Following device instructions, prepare strip and insert in glucometer

Read test results from the glucometer

Properly dispose of the test strip and lancet

3. Identify factors that may cause false glucometer readings. *p. 354*

Not using device according to manufacturer's instructions

Not matching code numbers to device and strip

Allowing alcohol to mix with blood

Using expired test strips

Placing a second drop of blood with the first

Not following manufacturer's recommendations for unit calibration

SUPPLEMENTAL INFORMATION

DIABETES MELLITUS

Glucose is an important body energy source. It is stored in the liver and at other sites and is transported from the blood stream into the body's cells with the help of insulin. The normal range for blood glucose is 80 to 120 mg/dL. If insulin production is abnormally low, the blood glucose level will rise above normal. If insulin production is high or the diabetic patient has injected insulin without adequate carbohydrate intake, the blood glucose level may drop dangerously low.

Diabetes mellitus is a very common disease with two different categories, type I and type II. Type I diabetes is a serious disease caused by inadequate insulin production by the pancreas. Type I diabetes is controlled by insulin injection and controlled diet. However, variations in volume or strength of insulin injected, patient activity, other diseases, or carbohydrate intake may lead to dangerously low or high blood sugar levels. Type II is a less severe adult onset diabetes that can often be controlled by diet and/or oral medication.

Diabetic ketoacidosis begins as low insulin levels prevent adequate glucose from entering the body cells. Glucose remains in the blood, and levels there begin to rise. The glucose spills into the urine and takes with it body water. The cells are without glucose for normal metabolism and rely on less efficient ways to obtain energy. The result is an acidosis due to the accumulation of acetones and ketones.

The onset of signs and symptoms of diabetic acidosis is slow, usually from 12 to 24 hours. The patient will display thirst, frequent urination, excessive hunger, and a general ill feeling. In later stages, the patient may display a sweet, fruity breath and deep, rapid respiration. Glucose levels will be elevated up to 300 to 600 mg/dL.

Acute hypoglycemia is a rapid onset emergency. The patient has taken too much insulin or has not eaten after insulin administration. The insulin rapidly moves the available blood glucose into the body cells, and the blood glucose level drops very low. The body cells, especially those of the brain, then become starved for glucose and may sustain serious injury.

Hypoglycemia presents rapidly with restlessness, impatience, drastic changes in behavior, rage, bizarre behavior, seizures, and coma. Blood glucose levels are low, usually well below 80 mg/dL.

Field glucose level determination can be very helpful in differentiating between acute hypoglycemia and diabetic ketoacidosis. Additionally, other patients such as the chronic alcoholic and the malnourished may be hypoglycemic.

CONTENT SELF-EVALUATION

MULTIPLE CHOICE

_____ **1.** The major criteria used to identify the need for determining the glucose level is a(n))
  A. history of diabetes.
  B. medic alert tag.
  C. history of chronic alcohol abuse.
  D. altered mental status.
  E. cool and clammy skin.

_____ **2.** When using the blood glucose determination device, an EMT-Intermediate should be sure the alcohol is still damp when the skin is lanced. This will help the blood distribute evenly over the test strip.
  A. True
  B. False

_____ **3.** The normal range of blood glucose is
  A. 20 to 40 mg/dL.
  B. 40 to 60 mg/dL.
  C. 60 to 80 mg/dL.
  D. 80 to 120 mg/dL.
  E. 120 to 200 mg/dL.

_____ **4.** The patient who has a history of diabetes, has administered insulin two hours earlier, has not eaten, and is displaying bizarre behavior is most likely to have as glucose level of
  A. 20 to 45 mg/dL.
  B. 80 to 100 mg/dL.
  C. 120 to 200 mg/dL.
  D. 200 to 300 mg/dL.
  E. none of the above

_____ **5.** Which of the following is a sign of diabetic ketoacidosis?
  A. thirst
  B. hunger
  C. frequent urination
  D. malaise
  E. all of the above

SPECIAL PROJECT

Place the following steps of blood glucose determination in the proper order.

6. _____ **A.** Read test results from the glucometer

7. _____ **B.** Follow universal precautions (don gloves)

8. _____ **C.** Lance the patient's finger and obtain a drop of blood

9. _____ **D.** Touch the blood drop to the target area of the test strip

10. _____ **E.** Cleanse the site with alcohol and allow time for complete evaporation

11. _____ **F.** Remove the test strip from container and check its expiration date

12. _____ **G.** Locate an appropriate fingerstick site

13. _____ **H.** Following device instructions, prepare the strip, and insert in the glucometer

14. _____ **I.** Properly dispose of the test strip and lancet

APPENDIX III

PHARMACOLOGY FOR THE EMT-INTERMEDIATE

APPENDIX III OBJECTIVES

After reading this appendix, you should be able to do the following:

1. **Define the following terms.** *pp. 355–360*

   Pharmacology—study of drugs and their effects on the human body

   Drug—chemical agent used in the diagnosis, treatment, or prevention of disease

   Pharmacokinetics—study of how drugs enter the body, reach their site of action, and are eventually eliminated

2. **List four drug sources and give an example of a drug derived from each source.** *p. 356*

   Plant—atropine (used in the treatment of heart blocks and bradycardia)

   Animal—insulin (extracted from the pancreas of cattle; used to treat diabetes)

   Mineral—sodium bicarbonate (used to combat metabolic acidosis in the cardiac arrest patient)

   Synthetic—lidocaine (used to treat cardiac dysrhythmia)

3. **Name three federal legislative acts that regulate drugs.** *p. 356*

   Federal Food, Drug, and Cosmetic Act of 1938—requires packagers to list the ingredients on foods and medications

   Harrison Narcotic Act—regulates the sale, importation, and manufacture of the opium plant and its derivatives

   Controlled Substances Act—regulates addictive drugs and defines the five schedules of controlled substances

4. **List the five addictive drug schedules and give an example of a medication from each.** *pp. 356–357*

   Schedule I—drugs that have a high potential for abuse and have no accepted medical indications; example: heroin

   Schedule II—drugs that have a high potential for abuse, but also have accepted medical indications; examples: morphine and meperidine

   Schedule III—drugs that have a reduced potential for abuse and accepted medication indications; examples: acetaminophen with codeine

   Schedule IV—drugs that have a low potential for abuse, but may cause a physical or psychological dependence; example: diazepam (Valium)

   Schedule V—drugs that have a low potential for abuse, yet contain small quantities of narcotics; examples: several types of cough medications

5. **List four names that can be used to identify a drug.** *p. 357*

   Chemical name
   Generic name
   Trade name
   Official name

6. Describe three common drug references and know how to find a medication in one of these references. *p. 357*

AMA drug evaluations—provides drug information on groups of drugs, including their recommended dosages, side effects, indications, and contraindications

Physicians' Desk Reference (PDR)—compilation of manufacturers' drug information on the most current drugs on the market; contains photographs showing the actual size, shape, and color of many of drugs; published yearly

Drug inserts—accompany most drugs and supply the manufacturer recommendations for use and other data

7. List several examples of both liquid and solid drugs. *pp. 357–359*

Liquids

Solutions—preparations in which the drugs are dissolved in a solvent, usually water; example: normal saline

Tinctures—drug preparations in which the drug was extracted chemically with the use of alcohol; example: tincture of iodine

Suspensions—drugs that do not dissolve in the solvent but are instead suspended in solution and will separate if not shaken frequently; example: amoxicillin

Spirits—volatile chemicals dissolved in alcohol; example: spirits of ammonia

Emulsions—mixtures of an oil substance and a solvent; do not dissolve well and must be shaken before administration

Elixirs—preparations that contain a drug in alcohol with an added flavoring; example: Tylenol elixir

Syrups—drugs mixed with sugar, water, and flavoring; example: cough syrup

Solids

Pills—drugs shaped for easy swallowing; example: vitamins

Powders—drugs in powder form, usually intended for mixing with another agent

Capsules—gelatin containers filled with a drug powder; drug released as gelatin dissolves in the intestinal tract; example: dalmane

Tablets—pressed powders shaped in an easy-to-swallow form; example: aspirin

Suppositories—drugs mixed with a base that dissolves at body temperature; placed rectally or vaginally and absorbed by surrounding tissues

8. Define "parenteral drugs." *p. 358*

Medications introduced through routes other than the digestive system, such as intravenous, intramuscular, and subcutaneous; the majority of EMS drugs

9. Define the following terms. *p. 358*

Ampule—glass or plastic single-dose container that must be broken to obtain and use the drug

Vial—single- or multi-dose container that is sealed with a rubber cap; drug obtained by withdrawing it with a needle and a syringe

Prefilled syringe—single-dose preloaded administration device; can be used rapidly and is common in EMS

10. Define important pharmacological terminology. *pp. 359–360*

Antagonism—opposition between the actions of two or more drugs

Bolus—single, often large, dose of medication

Contraindications—medical or physiological reasons for not using a drug

Cumulative action—result of administering several small doses and achieving an increasing effect, usually due to buildup of the drug in the blood

Depressant—medication that decreases a bodily function or activity

Habituation—psychological or physiological dependence on a drug

Hypersensitivity—exaggerated reactivity to a drug or other foreign substance

Idiosyncrasy—individual reaction to a drug that is very different from what is expected

Indication—medical condition for which the drug has a proven therapeutic value

Potentiation—enhancement of the effects on one drug by the administration of another

Refractory—condition in which a drug fails to provide the therapeutic action desired for the patient

Side effects—unavoidable and undesirable effects of a drug even in therapeutic doses

Stimulant—drug that increases a bodily function or activity

Synergism—combination of two drugs that together perform better than the sum of their isolated effects

Therapeutic action—intended action of a drug

Tolerance—reduction in the obtained effects of a dosage of a drug over time, thus requiring larger dosages to achieve the same effect

11. Define a drug's mechanism of action. *p. 360*

Chain of biochemical events that eventually lead to the physiological changes desired

12. List four factors that influence the concentration of a drug at its site of action. *pp. 360–362*

Absorption—entrance of the drug into the cardiovascular system

Distribution—movement of the drug to the site where it is to be used

Biotransformation—conversion of the drug into its active form

Elimination—withdrawal of the drug from the cardiovascular system and the removal of the drug from the body

13. List factors that slow drug absorption and factors that enhance it. *p. 361*

Factors that slow absorption—shock, acidosis, and peripheral vasoconstriction due to hypothermia

Factors that enhance absorption—peripheral vasodilation, as caused by fever, hyperthermia, or other conditions that increase the blood supply at the injection site

14. Define "blood barrier." *p. 361*

Mechanism that isolates the brain tissue from the bloodstream and selectively allows a limited number of compounds into the brain

15. Define "metric system." *p. 363*

System of measurement for mass, length, and volume; uses the decimal system (each unit is 10 times larger—or $\frac{1}{10}$ as large—as the next); basic units include grams, meters, and liters

16. Demonstrate the ability to do routine calculations and conversions using the metric system. *pp. 363–367*

See mathematical examples in Intermediate Emergency Care.

17. Be able to calculate any given drug dose for all medications used in your EMS system. *pp. 363–367*

See mathematical examples in Intermediate Emergency Care.

18. List ten routes of medication administration. *pp. 368–369*

Parenteral routes—intradermal, transdermal, subcutaneous, intramuscular, intravenous, endotracheal, intraosseus, inhalation, sublingual, intracardiac

Enteral routes—sublingual, oral, rectal

19. Identify the steps in administering an intravenous drug. *p. 371*

Follow universal precautions

Confirm indications for the drug and repeat orders back to the physician

Inspect medication for expiration, concentration, and any signs of contamination

Remove end caps and screw the drug cartridge into the syringe

Invert the syringe and expel any air and extra fluid

Select an appropriate injection site

Cleanse the injection site with alcohol

Insert the syringe needle into injection port

Pinch the IV tubing above injection site

Inject the drug slowly

Remove the syringe and place it in sharps container

Flush the IV line and open drip valve to flush line

Record the time and dosage administered

Monitor patient for signs of adverse reaction

20. Describe the administration of a drug via the intramuscular route. *pp. 373–375*

Equipment

Protective gloves and sharps container

Glucagon vial combination

3-mL syringe with 19–21 gauge 1–1$\frac{1}{2}$-inch needle

Alcohol wipes

Procedure (*Note:* Intramuscular route is used when other routes, such as IV, are not available. Absorption is slow, usually 10–30 minutes.)

Confirm the indications and physician orders for glucagon

Verify the correct drug, its concentration, expiration date, and sterile condition

Explain procedure to the patient and rule out possible drug allergy

Remove the cap from the two vials and clean their tops with alcohol

Inject 1 mL of air into the vial of solution and withdraw the solution

Inject the solution into the other vial, shake gently, and withdraw the solution

Hold the syringe up, tap it to move the bubbles up, then expel the air and excess drug

Don protective gloves

Locate the deltoid or other site and cleanse with alcohol, allowing the alcohol to dry

Stretch the skin and then displace it to one side or down one inch (Z-track)

Pull back on the plunger and, if no blood is returned, inject the drug

Wait 10 seconds, then remove the needle

Dispose of the needle and syringe properly and document the administration

Cover the site with an alcohol swab and massage it gently

21. Identify the signs, symptoms, and care of the patient who is experiencing anaphylaxis. *p. 376*

Signs and symptoms—dyspnea, wheezing, stridor, hypotension

Patient care—use of general shock care, including administration of oxygen, IV fluids, and 1:1,000 epinephrine

22. Explain and demonstrate subcutaneous injection. *pp. 376–379*

Equipment

Protective gloves and sharps container

1-mL syringe with 25-gauge, $\frac{5}{8}$-inch needle

Alcohol wipes

Epinephrine 1:1,000 ampule (1 mg in 1 mL)

Procedure (*Note:* This route provides a slow, sustained drug absorption causing minimal tissue trauma and carries limited risk of injection into blood vessels or nerves.)

Confirm the indications and physician order for epinephrine 1:1,000

Verify the correct drug, its concentration, expiration date, and sterile condition

Explain the procedure to the patient and rule out any drug allergy

Shake the ampule to empty neck of fluid

Wrap the ampule neck with a gauze 4 × 4 and break it

Invert the ampule, insert syringe, and withdraw the drug

Hold the syringe up, tap it to move bubbles up, then expel bubbles and excess drug

Don protective gloves

Locate the deltoid or other site and cleanse with alcohol, allowing the alcohol to dry

Pinch the skin up and insert the needle at a 45-degree angle, bevel up, into fatty tissue

Withdraw the plunger and, if no blood returns, inject the drug

Dispose of the needle and syringe properly and document the administration

Cover the site with an alcohol swab and massage it gently

23. Discuss the assessment and care of the patient who requires nebulized medications. *pp. 380–383*

Equipment

Oxygen tank and regulator

Small-volume nebulizer and mouthpiece kit

Sterile saline for dilution

Medication—albuterol, isoetharine, metaproterenol

Procedure (*Note:* Patients who may require nebulized medication will most commonly present with dyspnea as their chief complaint. Additionally, they may display tachycardia, accessory muscle usage, and wheezing. They will also identify a history of asthma, chronic bronchitis, or emphysema.)

Confirm the indications and physician orders for nebulized medication

Verify the correct drug, its concentration, expiration date, and sterile condition

Explain the procedure to the patient and rule out a drug allergy

Determine the patient's pulse and respiration rates

Auscultate both lung fields

Assemble oxygen tank, regulator, and nebulizer kit

Place medication into the nebulizer cup, and attach the oxygen tubing to the nebulizer

Set the oxygen flow to 8–10 liters per minute and attach the mouthpiece

Have the patient breath normally through the nebulizer mouthpiece

Record the time and dosage administered

Recheck the pulse, respirations, and auscultate the lung fields

Closely monitor the patient and document the pre- and post-treatment findings

24. Explain the indications and procedure for performing intraosseous medication administration. *pp. 383-386*

Indications—useful in children under age 5 when an intravenous line cannot otherwise be established

Contraindications—fractured bone or distal to a fractured bone

Equipment

Medication/intravenous fluid

Syringe

Intraosseous needle or 16–18 gauge spinal needle

Povidine iodine preparation

Procedure (*Note:* Fluids and medications administered through the bone marrow cavity can be rapidly introduced into the patient's blood stream.)

Confirm the indications and physician orders for intraosseous medication or fluid administration

Prepare necessary equipment and don gloves

Assure the drug/fluid is correct, not contaminated, or expired

Explain the procedure to the patient

Locate the anterior tibial tuberosity and choose a location site about 3 cm below this site

Prepare the area with povidine iodine, using a circular motion

Replace gloves with sterile gloves

Insert the needle at a right angle to the bone surface, using firm pressure until you feel the needle pop through the bone

Place the syringe on the needle and attempt to aspirate a small amount of bone marrow

If the needle stands on its own and if you can aspirate bone marrow, connect the IV line

Administer the medication or fluid (no more than 20 mL/kg at a time)

Remove the syringe and dispose of it properly

Monitor the patient for medication effectiveness and any side effects

Secure the intraosseous needle firmly in position, and protect from movement during transport

25. Explain and demonstrate the procedure for administering drugs via the endotracheal tube. *p. 386*

Indications—useful in intubated patients when (1) an intravenous line has not yet been established and (2) time is of the essence

Procedure

Secure the airway using an endotracheal tube as presented in Appendix I

Confirm the indications and medical control physical order for the drug

Prepare the medication syringe

Don sterile gloves, eye protection, and mask

Assure the drug/fluid is correct, not contaminated, or expired

Hyperventilate the patient

Remove the bag-valve-mask unit and forcefully inject the medication down the tube

Replace the bag-valve-mask unit and resume ventilation

Monitor the patient for effectiveness of the medication and any side effects

MULTIPLE CHOICE

_____ **1.** Which of the following is <u>not</u> a common source of drugs?
    A. plants
    B. minerals
    C. animals
    D. pharmacokinetics
    E. synthetics

_____ **2.** Which of the following is the origin of the drug lidocaine?
    A. plant
    B. mineral
    C. synthetic
    D. animal
    E. none of the above

_____ **3.** Under which schedule of medications do meperidine (Demerol) and morphine fall?
    A. Schedule I
    B. Schedule II
    C. Schedule III
    D. Schedule IV
    E. Schedule V

_____ **4.** The federal agency that bears primary responsibility for enforcement of the Controlled Substances Act is the
    A. Federal Bureau of Investigation.
    B. Division of Narcotic Enforcement.
    C. Drug Enforcement Agency.
    D. Harrison Narcotic and Controlled Substances Commission.
    E. Food and Drug Administration.

_____ **5.** Demerol HCL is an example of a drug's
    A. chemical name
    B. generic name
    C. trade name
    D. official name
    E. schedule name

_____ **6.** In which of the following references for drugs might an EMT-Intermediate find photographs of drugs to assist in their identification?
    A. AMA drug evaluations
    B. _Physicians' Desk Reference_
    C. Manufacturer drug inserts
    D. _Prehospital Emergency Pharmacology_
    E. all of the above

_____ **7.** Dextrose 5% in water (D_5W) is an example of a drug form known as a(n)
    A. solution.
    B. tincture.
    C. suspension.
    D. spirit.
    E. elixir.

_____ **8.** In prehospital emergency medicine, most drugs are supplied as
    A. ampules.
    B. single-dose vials.
    C. prefilled syringes.
    D. multi-dose vials.
    E. suspended and bagged solutions.

_____ **9.** The characteristic action of a drug that is unique to an individual is called
    A. idiosyncrasy.
    B. cumulative.
    C. refractory.
    D. synergism.
    E. uptoward.

_____ **10.** The process in which two drugs, administered in combination, produce a greater effect than the sum of their isolated effects, is known as
    A. idiosyncrasy.
    B. synergism.
    C. hypersensitivity.
    D. uptoward reaction.
    E. potentiation.

_____ **11.** The expected and intended action of a drug is referred to as its
  A. cumulative action.
  B. indication.
  C. therapeutic action.
  D. tolerance.
  E. design factor.

_____ **12.** The type of drug that binds to a receptor and causes the expected response is called an antagonist.
  A. True
  B. False

_____ **13.** Which of the following lists metric prefixes in order from smallest to largest?
  A. milli, kilo, centi
  B. milli, centi, kilo
  C. centi, milli, kilo
  D. kilo, centi, milli
  E. centi, kilo, milli

_____ **14.** The route of administration that permits a medication to be absorbed through the skin is
  A. intradermal.
  B. subcutaneous.
  C. intramuscular.
  D. oral.
  E. none of the above

_____ **15.** The most common route for the administration of drugs for emergency medical service is via the
  A. intramuscular route.
  B. intravenous route.
  C. subcutaneous route.
  D. oral route.
  E. sublingual route.

_____ **16.** It is advantageous to leave a small bubble of air at the top of the syringe because you can then watch your medication as it travels through the IV lines and into the patient.
  A. True
  B. False

_____ **17.** It is very safe to administer 50% dextrose in water (D_5W) because it closely matches the normal concentration of body fluid.
  A. True
  B. False

_____ **18.** Anaphylaxis occurs as a result of
  A. low blood pressure.
  B. excitement and hyperventilation.
  C. tissue swelling.
  D. massive release of histamine.
  E. none of the above

_____ **19.** The concentration of epinephrine used for subcutaneous injection is
  A. 1 gm/mL.
  B. 100 mg/mL.
  C. 10 mg/mL.
  D. 1:10,000.
  E. 1:1,000.

_____ **20.** The angle at which the needle for subcutaneous injection should be injected is
  A. 25 degrees.
  B. 35 degrees.
  C. 45 degrees.
  D. 60 degrees.
  E. 90 degrees.

_____ **21.** Factors that determine how well a subcutaneous drug will be absorbed include
  A. cardiovascular and fluid status.
  B. physical build and age.
  C. condition of the subcutaneous tissue.
  D. injection site and EMT-Intermediate skills.
  E. all of the above

_____ **22.** Medical control orders you to assist an anaphylaxis patient in administering his or her epinephrine by autoinjector. You should remove the protective cap and push the device against the thigh until it automatically injects the drug.
  A. True
  B. False

_____ **23.** What is the maximum volume of fluid to be run through an intraosseous site at a time?
  A. 5 mL/kg.
  B. 10 mL/kg.
  C. 20 mL/kg.
  D. 25 mL/kg.
  E. 40 mL/kg.

_____ **24.** When compared to intravenous doses, how much greater are doses of medication administered via the endotracheal route?
  A. 2–2.5 times as large.
  B. 3 times as large.
  C. 5 times as large.
  D. 10 times as large.
  E. 10–15 times as large.

_____ **25.** Which of the following drugs would an EMT-Intermediate use to induce vomiting in cases of a poisoning?
  A. sodium bicarbonate
  B. thiamin
  C. atropine sulfate
  D. syrup of ipecac
  E. Nitro Stat

SPECIAL PROJECT

Study the photographs on the steps in the procedure for subcutaneous administration on the next page. For each of the eight steps, write a brief caption.

A. _____

B. _____

C. _____

D. _____

E. _____

F. _____

G. _____

H. _____

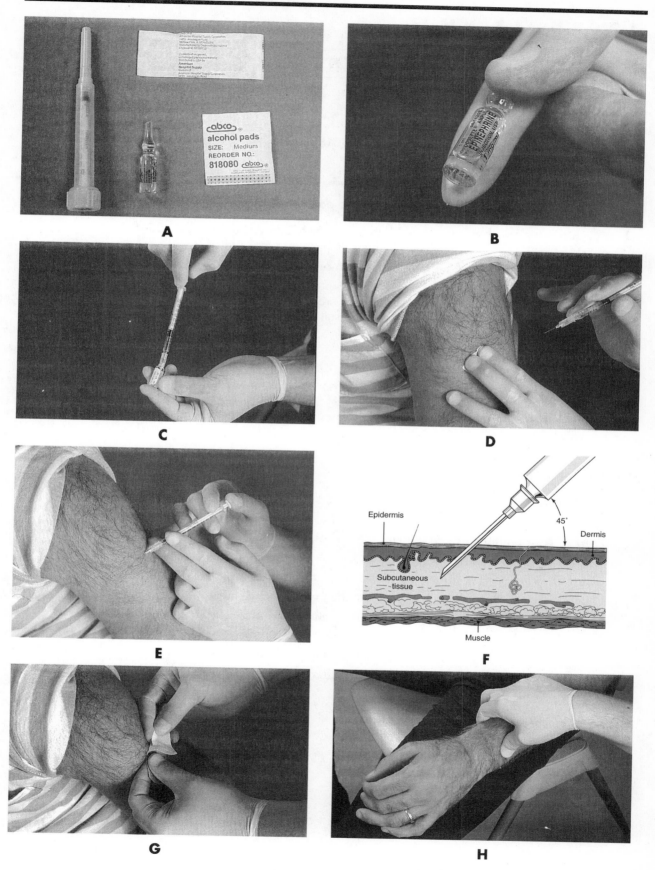

A

B

C

D

E

F

Epidermis
45°
Dermis
Subcutaneous tissue
Muscle

G

H

APPENDIX IV

ACCESSING INDWELLING CATHETERS

APPENDIX IV OBJECTIVES

After reading this appendix, you should be able to do the following:

1. **Explain why and how you would access indwelling catheters.** *pp. 408–410*

   Reasons for use—can utilize previously established venous access (the Hickman indwelling catheter) to obtain blood, administer medications, and provide fluid resuscitation

   Access—look for a long tube surgically inserted into the right atrium; used to avoid repetitive venipuncture in patients with chronic disease requiring frequent IV medication; access site usually covered with a dressing and a plug in the distal end (*Note:* Use this method of venous access only for emergencies.)

Equipment

Standard IV setup

30 mL vial of bacteriostatic saline

Syringes: 20 mL, 5 mL, 3 mL, and 18-gauge needle

Alcohol or Betadine wipes

Protective eyewear and sterile gloves

Latex-covered hemostat

Procedure

Confirm the patient's condition and the need to access the indwelling catheter

Prepare your equipment and explain the process to your patient

Wash your hands, don sterile gloves, and draw up 3 mL of normal saline

Clamp the catheter just above the dressings, and remove the tape from the Luer lock

Clean the connection port, allow it to dry, then remove and discard the intermittent infusion device

Connect a 5-mL syringe, release the clamp, withdraw 5 mL of fluid, and discard

Reattach the clamp, connect the 3-mL syringe, and flush the tube

Connect the IV tubing to the catheter and adjust the infusion rate

Monitor the IV and site as you would any other

MULTIPLE CHOICE

_____ **1.** In emergency situations, an indwelling catheter gives an EMT-Intermediate an opportunity to conduct all the following except

    A. draw blood.

    B. administer medications.

    C. establish numerous venipunctures.

    D. immediately access a patient's circulation.

    E. perform fluid resuscitation.

_____ **2.** Indwelling catheters are placed for all of the following reasons except

    A. gastrointestinal disorders.

    B. debilitating diseases.

    C. cancer treatment.

    D. long-term antibiotic therapy.

    E. routine access to the vascular system.

_____ **3.** Patients with indwelling catheters use it for self-administration of medications.

    A. True

    B. False

_____ **4.** The step that comes first in establishing IV access on a patient with an indwelling catheter is

    A. donning sterile gloves.

    B. explaining the process to the patient.

    C. confirming the need for use of a Hickman.

    D. preparing the equipment.

_____ **5.** All of the following are special precautions when accessing an indwelling catheter except

    A. maintaining sterile technique as much as possible.

    B. preventing air from entering the catheter.

    C. using hemostats with "teeth."

    D. clamping the catheter whenever the end is exposed.

    E. avoiding use of anything sharp

APPENDIX V

PULSE OXIMETRY

APPENDIX V OBJECTIVES

After reading this appendix, you should be able to do the following:

1. Describe the operation of the pulse oximeter. *pp. 411–412*

Consists of a probe, an electrical black box, and a display unit

Probe—senses the colors of light absorbed by the tissue of a finger, an earlobe, or other distal tissue

Black box—analyzes the signal received by the probe and determines the ratio of color absorbed by hemoglobin with oxygen and hemoglobin without; converts the ratio to oxygen saturation

Display unit—shows oxygen saturation along with pulse rate and an indicator identifying the strength or relative accuracy of the signal

2. Explain the operation of the pulse oximeter and its use in prehospital care. *pp. 413–414*

Operation—a non-invasive device that evaluates the effectiveness of the respiratory and cardiovascular systems in delivering oxygenated blood to the distal circulation

Steps in use—attached to finger or other distal tissue, unit turned on, reading delivered in 8 to 10 seconds, kept in use throughout patient care as a tool for evaluating effectiveness of interventions (*Note:* The normal reading will be between 96 and 100 percent. This reading is consistent with a normally functioning cardiorespiratory system. A reading between 90 and 95 percent reflects possible hypoxia, shock, or respiratory compromise. Such a reading should cause you to provide supplemental oxygen and watch for any further deterioration. A reading below 90 percent suggests severe hypoxia and requires aggressive respiratory support. Provide 100 percent oxygen, consider bag-valve-masking the patient, and consider endotracheal intubation.)

3. Identify the circumstances that can affect pulse oximeter readings. *pp. 415–418*

Chronic low-oxygen saturation

Chronic obstructive pulmonary disease—may cause a chronic low saturation (*Note:* In chronic bronchitis and emphysema, the patient may retain carbon dioxide and more residual air than healthier patients. This decreases the oxygen saturation over time, a condition to which the patient adjusts. Use your oximetry reading to titrate oxygen administration.)

High altitude—reduces the pressure that drives the oxygen into the hemoglobin (*Note:* If movement to a higher altitude occurs gradually or continues over a long time, the patient will adjust by producing more red blood cells. A lower saturation reading would be expected at high altitude, and for someone who lived there it would be normal. For someone who just arrived at a high altitude from sea level, however, such a reading would reflect an oxygen deficit.)

False readings

Carbon monoxide—replaces oxygen on the hemoglobin molecule and prevents oxygen delivery to the cells (*Note:* The oximeter reads the color of the carbon monoxide similarly to oxygen, giving a falsely high reading. You must rule out the possibility of carbon monoxide poisoning before putting full faith in the pulse oximetry reading.)

Nitroglycerin and sulfa drugs—may affect readings if administered at high doses and over relatively long times; some ingested or inhaled toxins may also affect readings (*Note:* These circumstances are relatively rare and will only alter the reading slightly.)

Low-flow states

Cold exposure—can reduce the circulation through the distal tissue, reducing the distal arterial pulse and the quality of oximetry signal (*Note:* In cold environments, warm the skin before probe placement and keep the area warm during your assessment, care, and transport to assure an accurate reading.)

Hypovolemia—can result in poor peripheral pulses and erratic pulse oximeter readings (*Note:* If you are caring for a patient who may be going into or in hypovolemic shock and the pulse oximeter is reading erratically, consider it a warning sign.)

CONTENT SELF-EVALUATION

MULTIPLE CHOICE

_____ **1.** A drop in the oxygen saturation from 100 to 90 percent reflects a reduction in the oxygen carrying capacity of the blood of about

    A. 40 percent.
    B. 30 percent.
    C. 20 percent.
    D. 10 percent.
    E. less than 5 percent.

_____ **2.** The normal oxygen saturation reading for a pulse oximeter when applied to a patient without cardiovascular or respiratory problem is

    A. 85 to 90 percent.
    B. 91 to 95 percent.
    C. 96 to 100 percent.
    D. greater than 100 percent.
    E. none of the above

_____ **3.** What effect would you expect hypovolemia or cold exposure to have on your pulse oximeter readings?

    A. erratic readings
    B. false low reading
    C. false high readings
    D. no effect
    E. no reading at all

SPECIAL PROJECT

Match the letter of the reading you would most expect to find on a pulse oximeter for each of the conditions below.

    A. false high reading
    B. erratic reading
    C. correct but low reading

_____ **4.** emphysema

_____ **5.** cold exposure

_____ **6.** high altitude

_____ **7.** cigarette smoking

_____ **8.** hypovolemia

Workbook Answer Key

CHAPTER 1

ROLES AND RESPONSIBILITIES OF THE EMT-INTERMEDIATE

CONTENT SELF-EVALUATION

MULTIPLE CHOICE

1. B	**6.** E	**11.** A
2. A	**7.** B	**12.** E
3. B	**8.** C	**13.** D
4. E	**9.** A	**14.** D
5. C	**10.** D	**15.** A

DESCRIPTION

16. (at least 3)
- be mentally, physically, and emotionally prepared
- display practical skill mastery
- be aware of treatment protocols and general medical knowledge
- be aware of local geography
- be knowledgeable of communications operation
- be aware of support services
- have leadership qualities

17. (at least 5)
- size up and secure the scene
- determine resource needs
- patient assessment
- assign priorities of care
- communicate with crew members
- initiate basic and advanced life support
- assess effects of treatment
- communicate with Medical Control
- coordinate patient transport
- maintain rapport with patient, support agencies, and hospital personnel

18. (at least 5)
- self-confidence
- credibility
- inner strength
- assume control
- communication skills
- willing to make decisions
- willing to accept responsibilities
- knowledgeable about crew member capabilities

19. (at least 3)
- clean-cut
- responded promptly
- solution for everything
- remained calm
- skillful
- top quality care

20. (at least 3)
- case reviews
- videotapes
- cassette lectures
- in-hospital rotations in patient care areas
- field drills
- mobile classrooms that bring educational presentations to outlying squads
- self-study exercises and computer-aided instruction
- periodic "teaching days," in which a variety of topics are covered in lectures and presentations

SPECIAL PROJECT

The address for the National Registry of EMTs is:
6610 Busch Blvd.
P.O. Box 29233
Columbus, OH 43229
614-888-4484

CHAPTER 2

EMERGENCY MEDICAL SERVICES SYSTEMS

CONTENT SELF-EVALUATION

MULTIPLE CHOICE

1. A	**8.** B	**15.** A
2. A	**9.** C	**16.** E
3. C	**10.** B	**17.** E
4. B	**11.** A	**18.** D
5. A	**12.** E	**19.** A
6. B	**13.** E	
7. E	**14.** A	

SEQUENCING

20. A. 1, **B.** 4, **C.** 3, **D.** 2

DESCRIPTION

21. *Triage protocols (at least 1)*
- guidelines to determining what level of EMS response
- guidelines to determine where a particular patient will be sent
- guidelines to help physician make decisions involving patient flow through the EMS system

Treatment protocols (at least 2)
- guidelines for patient care
- direct orders by a physician (on-line)
- standing orders (off-line)

Transport protocols (at least 2)
- guidelines to determine mode of transport (air or ground)
- level of care determined by nature of illness or injury, patient condition, transport time

Transfer protocols (at least 1)
- guidelines for inter-hospital patient transports
- ensure patient travels to an appropriate facility

22. *EMT-Basic (at least 5)*
- CPR
- airway management
- hemorrhage control
- stabilization of fractures
- emergency childbirth

- basic extrication
- communication
- use of the pneumatic anti-shock garment
- automatic defibrillation (in some cases)

EMT-Intermediate (at least 2)
- skills of the EMT-Basic ■ other advanced skills
- use of the EOA or EGTA■ intravenous fluid therapy

EMT-Paramedic (at least 4)
- skills of the EMT-Basic
- skills of the EMT-Intermediate
- advanced patient assessment
- trauma management
- endotracheal intubation
- pharmacology and drug administration
- cardiology (monitoring, cardioversion, and defibrillation)
- other medical emergency care

23. **A.** Caller interrogation—asks standard questions.
    B. Prioritization of symptoms—determines level of response.
    C. Appropriate response—types of personnel, number of vehicles, mode of response.
    D. Lifesaving pre-arrival instructions—first aid techniques while units are responding.

SPECIAL PROJECT

Research—Basic Life Support
Hypothesis: You should formulate a theory to be proved or disproved. (for example: Correct instruction in blood pressure determination will improve student accuracy.)

Literature review:
magazines—*JEMS, Emergency,* etc.;
journals—*Annals of Emergency Medicine,* etc.;
textbooks—Basic level, Paramedic, etc.

Study methods: Your sample study method should be similar to this:

Had six EMTs take blood pressure readings on one another. They all used the same sphygmomanometer and stethoscope and applied the procedure in a quiet room. Each of the EMT's readings were compared with the average for each person on whom they took the readings. The EMTs repeated the experiment after the group received instruction on the correct procedures for determining blood pressure.

Conclusion: Your sample conclusion should be similar to this in wording:

During the first attempt to determine blood pressure, 70 percent of the readings were within the plus or minus 12 percent of the average blood pressure reading of the patient. Repeating the study after instruction increased the percentage of readings within 12 percent of average to 80 percent. A valid conclusion is that proper instruction in correct procedures significantly improves the accuracy of blood pressure readings.

CHAPTER 3

Medical-Legal Considerations of Emergency Care

CONTENT SELF-EVALUATION

MULTIPLE CHOICE

1. D	**5.** B	**9.** B
2. E	**6.** B	**10.** B
3. B	**7.** E	**11.** D
4. E	**8.** A	**12.** A

DESCRIPTION

13. Negligence is the failure of the EMT-Intermediate to meet the standard of care when he or she had the duty to act and when his or her actions contribute to the harm suffered by the patient.

    Res ipsa loquitur is a form of negligence in which the nature of the events suggest that the EMT-Intermediate caused harm to the patient. The burden to prove innocence becomes the responsibility of the EMT-Intermediate.

14.
    - The patient is unconscious.
    - The patient is unable to communicate.
    - The patient is mentally impaired.
    - The patient is a young child.

15.
    - The patient is an elderly, thin male.
    - He has a history of emphysema.
    - He is on 3 L of oxygen per minute vial nasal cannula.
    - He has a bedside nebulizer.
    - His respiratory rate is 6 and very shallow.
    - His pulse is weak and rapid.
    - The patient's daughter requested no resuscitation.
    - No valid DNR was found.
    - The patient's wife requested resuscitation.
    - The crew discussed DNR, and rejected the daughter's request.
    - Respiration was assisted via a bag-valve (BVM) unit.
    - Patient's color improved with mechanical ventilation.
    - An endotracheal tube was placed w/bilaterally equal breath sounds noted.
    - Pulse rate increased in rate and strength.

SPECIAL PROJECT
Answers will depend upon your state's requirements. Please confirm your answers with your instructor.

CHAPTER 4

MEDICAL TERMINOLOGY

MEDICAL TERM DISSECTION

	Prefix	Root	Suffix
1. myasthenia		muscle	weakness
2. cephalgia		head	pain
3. percuss	through	shake violently	
4. cyanosis		blue	condition
5. hyperflexion	over	bending	
6. pathology		disease	study
7. tachypnea	rapid	breathing	
8. rhinorrhea		nose	flow
9. dysuria	difficult	urination	
10. hypertrophy	over	nourishment	
11. osteocyte		bone	cell
12. hypoxemia	low	oxygen	blood
13. adrenal	toward	kidney	
14. hepatomegaly		liver	enlarged
15. abduct	away	guide	
16. otoscope		ear	examine
17. perinatal	around	birth	
18. antecubital	before	elbow	
19. dissect	twice	cut	
20. epicardium	above	heart	
21. postpartum	after	birth	
22. intervertebral	between	spinal bones	
23. neuroplasty		nerve	repair
24. hemothorax	blood	thorax	
25. polyphagia	frequent	eating	

COMMON MEDICAL ABBREVIATIONS

26. abd. — abdomen
27. ARDS — Adult Respiratory Distress Syndrome
28. ASHD — Atherosclerotic Heart Disease
29. AMA — Against Medical Advice
30. BBB — Bundle Branch Block
31. b.i.d. — twice per day
32. C/C — Chief Complaint
33. CHF — Congestive Heart Failure
34. COPD — Chronic Obstructive Pulmonary Disease
35. CSF — Cerebrospinal Fluid
36. Dx — diagnosis
37. DPT — Diphtheria Pertussis Tetanus Vaccine
38. ETOH — ethanol alcohol
39. fx — fracture
40. GSW — gunshot wound
41. GU — Genito-Urinary
42. Hct. — hematocrit
43. Hx — history
44. IPPB — Intermittent Positive Pressure Breathing
45. JVD — Jugular Vein Distension
46. MVA — Motor Vehicle Accident
47. NPO — nothing by mouth
48. PRN — as needed
49. pt. — patient
50. Rx — care or remedy
51. S/S — Signs and Symptoms
52. S.O.B. — Short of Breath
53. TKO — To Keep Open
54. wt. — weight
55. y.o. — years old

SPECIAL PROJECT

Use one of the medical dictionaries listed at the end of Chapter 4 in *Intermediate Emergency Care.*

CHAPTER 5

EMS COMMUNICATIONS

CONTENT SELF-EVALUATION

MULTIPLE CHOICE

1. C	**5.** B	**9.** D
2. B	**6.** C	**10.** E
3. C	**7.** A	**11.** A
4. D	**8.** E	**12.** E

SEQUENCING

13. A. 3, **B.** 4, **C.** 1, **D.** 2

DESCRIPTION

14. (any 2)
- establish technical standards for radio equipment
- approve radio protocols for EMS systems
- license and allocate radio frequencies
- monitor radio frequencies to assure appropriate usage
- check station licenses and station records
- license and regulate technical personnel who repair and operate equipment

15. (any 3)
- direct the appropriate vehicle to the appropriate address
- monitor and coordinate system communications
- obtain information necessary for the EMS response
- instruct the caller in first aid measures
- maintain records of the complete response

SPECIAL PROJECT

Your reports should include most of the following elements.

Radio message from the scene to medical control:
Unit 89 to Receiving Hospital

We are at the ball field treating a 13-year-old male who collapsed while playing baseball. He is currently unresponsive to all but painful stimuli, is cool to the touch and sweating profusely. Vitals are BP 136/98, pulse 92 and strong, respirations 24 and regular, and pupils equal and slow to react. ECG is showing normal sinus rhythm. No physical signs of trauma noted and past medical history is unknown. Oxygen is applied at 4 liters via nasal cannula. Expected ETA 20 minutes.

Follow-up radio message to medical control:
One IV in left forearm running TKO with NS. Patient now responding to verbal stimuli. Vitals BP 134/96, pulse 90 & strong, respirations 24, ECG—NSR. ETA, 10 minutes

Ambulance run report form:
Please review the next page and ensure that your form includes the appropriate information. Note that you should include most, if not all, of the information listed on the example form. If not, please review the narrative in the workbook and determine what you are missing. Ensure that no important details are left out of the report.

Date **Today's Date**	Emergency Medical Services Run Report	Run # **911**

Patient Information — **Service Information** — **Times**

Patient Information	Service Information	Times
Name: **Thompson, John**	Agency: **Unit 89**	Rcvd **15:15**
Address: **Unknown**	Location: **Ballfield**	Enrt **15:15**
City: St: Zip:	Call Origin: **Dispatch**	Scne **15:22**
Age: **13** Birth: / / Sex: [**M**][F]	Type: Emrg[**X**] Non[ ] Trnsfr[ ]	LvSn **15:40**
Nature of Call: **Person Collapsed**		ArHsp **15:57**
Chief Complaint: **Unconsciousness—possible heat exhaustion**		InSv **16:15**

Description of Current Problem:

The patient collapsed while playing baseball on a very hot, sunny

day. Pt. was found to be cool & diaphoretic, unresponsive to

verbal stimuli, and responsive to painful stimuli. Pupils were

normal in size but slow to react. Physical assessment reveals no

apparent signs of trauma or other medical problem

Medical Problems

Past		Present
[ ]	Cardiac	[ ]
[ ]	Stroke	[ ]
[ ]	Acute Abdomen	[ ]
[ ]	Diabetes	[ ]
[ ]	Psychiatric	[ ]
[ ]	Epilepsy	[ ]
[ ]	Drug/Alcohol	[ ]
[ ]	Poisoning	[ ]
[ ]	Allergy/Asthma	[ ]
[ ]	Syncope	[ ]
[ ]	Obstetrical	[ ]
[ ]	GYN	[ ]

Other:

Trauma Scr: **n/a**   Glascow: **6**

On Scene Care: **provided oxygen, removed**

patient from sun and heat. Attempted IV in right

forearm (unsuccessful) started IV in left

forearm w/ 16 ga NS – TKO

First Aid: **pillow was placed under head**

By Whom? **bystanders**

02 @ **4** L **15:25** Via **NC**	C-Collar **n/a** :	S-Immob. **n/a**	Stretcher **15:37**

Allergies/Meds: **Unknown**

Past Med Hx: **Unknown**

Time	Pulse		Resp.		BP S/D	LOC	ECG
15:27	R: **92**	[**X**][i]	R: **24**	[s][l]	**136/98**	[a][v][**X**][u]	**Normal Sinus Rhythm**
Care/Comments: **Pt. unresponsive to all but painful stimuli**							
15:37	R: **90**	[**X**][i]	R: **24**	[s][l]	**134/96**	[a][**X**][p][u]	**Normal Sinus Rhythm**
Care/Comments: **Pt. became responsive to verbal stimuli**							
15:45	R: **88**	[**X**][i]	R: **22**	[s][l]	**132/90**	[**X**][v][p][u]	**Normal Sinus Rhythm**
Care/Comments: **Pt. became fully conscious, alert, and oriented**							
:	R:	[r][i]	R:	[s][l]	/	[a][v][p][u]	
Care/Comments:							

Destination: **Receiving Hospital**	Personnel:	Certification
Reason:[ ]pt [**X**]Closest [ ]M.D. [ ]Other	1. **Your Name**	[P][**X**][O]
Contacted: [**X**]Radio [ ]Tele [ ]Direct	2. **Steve Phillips**	[P][**X**][O]
Ar Status: [**X**]Better [ ]UnC [ ]Worse	3. **n/a**	[P][E][O]

CHAPTER 6: PART I

GENERAL PATIENT ASSESSMENT AND INITIAL MANAGEMENT

CONTENT SELF-EVALUATION

MULTIPLE CHOICE

1. E	**4.** D	**7.** D
2. C	**5.** D	**8.** E
3. D	**6.** C	

SEQUENCING

9. A. 4, **B.** 5, **C.** 2, **D.** 3, **E.** 1, **F.** 6

10. A. 4, **B.** 2, **C.** 3, **D.** 1

11. *Information from the Dispatcher*
- type of medical emergency
- vehicle placement
- seriousness of the call
- skills and equipment needed
- best scene approach

12. *Information from scene survey*
- mechanism of injury/nature of illness
- scene hazards
- number of patients
- location of patients
- additional resources needed

SPECIAL PROJECT

Radio message from the scene to medical control:
Unit 21 to Medical Control. We are attending a male victim of a one-car accident. He was initially unconscious but is now conscious, alert, and oriented. He has a small contusion on his forehead and a small welt on his neck. He was stung by a bee and has had a previous allergic reaction. Vitals are BP 110/76, pulse 90 and strong, respirations 24, and O_2 saturation of 94%. There are wheezes audible and he is complaining of "a lump in the throat." He is on 12 L of O_2 via non-rebreather and has one IV of LR running TKO. A cervical collar has been applied and spinal immobilization is underway.

Follow-up radio message to Community Hospital:
Current vitals are BP 122/78, pulse 68 and strong, respirations 22 and regular, O_2 saturation 98%. Patient requests transport to Community Hospital.

CHAPTER 6: PART II

GENERAL PATIENT ASSESSMENT AND INITIAL MANAGEMENT

CONTENT SELF-EVALUATION

MULTIPLE CHOICE

13. B	**20.** D
14. A	**21.** C
15. E	**22.** C
16. B	**23.** D
17. A	**24.** B
18. C	**25.** A
19. D	

CHAPTER 7: PART I

AIRWAY MANAGEMENT AND VENTILATION

CONTENT SELF-EVALUATION

MULTIPLE CHOICE

1. B	**6.** D	**11.** B
2. A	**7.** E	**12.** D
3. C	**8.** C	**13.** D
4. C	**9.** E	**14.** E
5. C	**10.** A	**15.** E

LABEL THE DIAGRAM

16. A. Tonsil   **E.** Vocal Cords
     B. Tongue   **F.** Trachea
     C. Vallecula   **G.** Cricoid Cartilage
     D. Epiglottis   **H.** Esophagus

SPECIAL PROJECT

Airway Obstruction

1. ***Tongue*** In the absence of muscle tone, the relaxed tongue drops back in the larynx blocking the airway.
2. ***Foreign body*** An object, usually food, becomes lodged in the laryngopharynx and blocks the airway.
3. ***Trauma*** Trauma may disrupt the integrity of the airway thereby allowing it to collapse or physically blocking the airway. Additionally, loose teeth or blood clots may obstruct the airway.
4. ***Laryngeal edema or spasm*** Swelling of the laryngeal tissue may occlude the airway or spasm of the vocal cords may occur secondary to anaphylaxis, epiglottitis, or inhalation of harmful substances.
5. ***Aspiration*** The inhalation of teeth, dentures, blood, or vomitus may occlude the airway.

Normal Respiratory Values

	Inspired Air	Alveolar Air		
% Oxygen	21%	14%	PaO_2	80–100 Torr
% CO_2	0.04%	5%	$PaCO_2$	35–45 Torr

Normal Respiration Rate/Volumes

Infant 40 to 60   Child 18 to 24   Adult 12 to 20

Tidal Volume	500 mL
Alveolar Volume	350 mL
Dead Space Volume	150 mL
Minute Volume	4,500 mL

CHAPTER 7: PART II

AIRWAY MANAGEMENT AND VENTILATION

CONTENT SELF-EVALUATION

MULTIPLE CHOICE

17.	B	32.	E
18.	A	33.	A
19.	E	34.	E
20.	D	35.	B
21.	E	36.	E
22.	C	37.	A
23.	A	38.	C
24.	E	39.	A
25.	E	40.	A
26.	B	41.	B
27.	C	42.	C
28.	A	43.	D
29.	C	44.	E
30.	E	45.	A
31.	A	46.	D

SPECIAL PROJECT

Problem Solving—Airway Maintenance

What equipment would you prepare?

suction   tape   10 mL syringe
laryngoscope   stethoscope   water-soluble gel
stylet   endotracheal tube Magill forceps

How would you check your equipment?
Laryngoscope Check blade—bright white and non-flickering
Tube cuff Inflate with 10 mL—will it hold air?
One larger and one smaller tube available

What would you ask the ventilator to do prior to your attempt?
Hyperventilate the patient.

Identify the steps of the procedures you're about to attempt.
1. Fill syringe with 10–15 mL air.
2. Position the patient's head.
3. Grasp the handle in left hand.
4. Insert blade in right side of mouth.
5. Displace tongue to left.
6. Insert blade to epiglottis.
7. Lift laryngoscope along axis of handle.
8. Visualize the vocal folds and glottis.
9. Grasp tube and pass it between the cords.
10. Inflate the cuff and auscultate.

What actions would you take to ensure the tube is properly placed?
1. Visualize, with the laryngoscope, the tube passing through the vocal folds.
2. Check the depth of the tube against the mouth.
3. Auscultate all lung fields for bilaterally equal breath sounds.
4. Auscultate epigastrium for gurgling sounds.

What should you do if the tube is misplaced?
If the tube is placed in the esophagus, leave it in place, hyperventilate the patient and attempt to place another tube in the trachea. Reauscultate and assure the tube is properly placed.

CHAPTER 8: PART I

FLUIDS AND SHOCK

CONTENT SELF-EVALUATION

MULTIPLE CHOICE

1.	A	11.	C
2.	A	12.	A
3.	B	13.	E
4.	C	14.	B
5.	D	15.	E
6.	B	16.	C
7.	D	17.	B
8.	E	18.	B
9.	A	19.	C
10.	E	20.	D

SPECIAL PROJECT
A. 4.5%, **B.** 15%, **C.** 10.5%, **D.** 45%,

CHAPTER 8: PART II

FLUIDS AND SHOCK

CONTENT SELF-EVALUATION

MULTIPLE CHOICE

21.	E	29.	B
22.	D	30.	D
23.	B	31.	C
24.	D	32.	B
25.	B	33.	E
26.	D	34.	A
27.	C	35.	D
28.	A	36.	B

SPECIAL PROJECT
Analyzing Signs of Shock

Cool and clammy skin: Peripheral vasoconstriction reduces blood flow to the skin.

Agitation: Cerebral hypoxia due to reduced circulation to the brain and reduced levels of oxygen because of reduced efficiency of respiration or oxygen-carrying capability of the blood.

Rapid pulse: A cardiovascular compensatory mechanism to maintain blood pressure and perfusion when cardiac preload is reduced due to hypovolemia.

Dropping blood pressure: A late sign of shock occurring when compensatory mechanisms fail and the heart and arterial system cannot maintain blood pressure and circulation.

Ashen or cyanotic skin: As the body compensates for volume loss, it shunts blood from the skin and results in deoxygenation of the blood still within the skin and hence the ashen and cyanotic colors.

Analyzing Drops in Blood Pressure
Blood pressure drops late in the shock process because the compensatory mechanisms compensate for blood loss and maintain the blood pressure. This includes vasoconstriction, increased heart rate, and shunting of blood to the central organs only.

Appendix Answer Key

APPENDIX I

DEFIBRILLATION

CONTENT SELF-EVALUATION

MULTIPLE CHOICE

1. A	6. B	10. A
2. D	7. C	11. E
3. B	8. B	12. E
4. A	9. B	13. C
5. E		

APPENDIX II

BLOOD GLUCOSE DETERMINATION

CONTENT SELF-EVALUATION

MULTIPLE CHOICE

1. D	3. D	5. E
2. B	4. A	

SPECIAL PROJECT

6. B	9. F	12. H
7. G	10. C	13. A
8. E	11. D	14. I

APPENDIX III

EMERGENCY PHARMACOLOGY FOR THE EMT-INTERMEDIATE

CONTENT SELF-EVALUATION

MULTIPLE CHOICE

1. D	10. B	19. E
2. C	11. C	20. C
3. B	12. A	21. E
4. C	13. B	22. A
5. C	14. E	23. C
6. B	15. B	24. A
7. A	16. B	25. D
8. C	17. B	
9. A	18. D	

SPECIAL PROJECT

Ask a classmate, your instructor, or an EMT-Intermediate in your EMS system to critique your captions for accuracy and clarity.

APPENDIX IV

ACCESSING INDWELLING CATHETERS

CONTENT SELF-EVALUATION

MULTIPLE CHOICE

1. C	3. A	5. C
2. E	4. C	

APPENDIX V

PULSE OXIMETRY

CONTENT SELF-EVALUATION

MULTIPLE CHOICE

1. A	2. C	3. A

SPECIAL PROJECT

4. C	6. C	8. B
5. C	7. A	

NATIONAL REGISTRY OF EMTS EMT-INTERMEDIATE PRACTICAL EXAMINATIONS

1. PATIENT ASSESSMENT/MANAGEMENT

2. VENTILATORY MANAGEMENT (ET)

3. VENTILATORY MANAGEMENT (EOA)

4. INTRAVENOUS THERAPY

5. SPINAL IMMOBILIZATION (SEATED PATIENT)

6. BLEEDING—WOUNDS—SHOCK

7. LONG BONE IMMOBILIZATION

8. TRACTION SPLINTING

9. SPINAL IMMOBILIZATION (LYING PATIENT)

National Registry of Emergency Medical Technicians
Advanced Level Practical Examination

PATIENT ASSESSMENT/MANAGEMENT

Candidate: _____   Examiner: _____
Date: _____   Signature: _____
Scenario# _____   Time Start: _____ Time End: _____

		Possible Points	Points Awarded
PRIMARY SURVEY/RESUSCITATION			
Takes or verbalizes infection control precautions		1	
Airway with C-Spine Control	Takes or directs manual in-line immobilization of head (1 point) Opens and assesses airway (1 point) Inserts adjunct (1 point)	3	
Breathing	Assesses breathing (1 point) Initiates appropriate oxygen therapy (1 point) Assures adequate ventilation of patient (1 point) Manages any injury which may compromise breathing/ventilation (1 point)	4	

Circulation	Checks pulse (1 point)
	Assesses peripheral perfusion (1 point)
	   [checks either skin color, temperature, or capillary refill]
	Assesses for and controls major bleeding if present (1 point)
	Takes vital signs (1 point)
	Verbalizes application of or consideration for PASG (1 point)
	   [candidate must assess body parts to be enclosed prior to application]
		5	

	Volume replacement [usually deferred until patient loaded]
	   –Initiates first IV line (1 point)
	   –Initiates second IV line (1 point)
	   –Selects appropriate catheters (1 point)
	   –Selects appropriate IV solutions and administration sets (1 point)
	   –Infuses at appropriate rate (1 point)
		5	

Disability	Performs mini-neuro assessment: AVPU (1 point) Applies cervical collar (1 point)	2	
Expose	Removes clothing	1	
Status	Calls for immediate transport of the patient when indicated	1	
	PRIMARY SURVEY/RESUSCITATION SUB-TOTAL	22	

	NOTE: Areas denoted by "**" may be integrated within sequence of Primary Survey		
SECONDARY SURVEY			
Head	Inspects mouth**, nose**, and assesses facial area (1 point) Inspects and palpates scalp and ears (1 point) Checks eyes: PEARRL** (1 point)	3	
Neck**	Checks position of trachea (1 point) Checks jugular veins (1 point) Palpates cervical spine (1 point)	3	
Chest**	Inspects chest (1 point) Palpates chest (1 point) Auscultates chest (1 point)	3	
Abdomen/Pelvis**	Inspects and palpates abdomen (1 point) Assesses pelvis (1 point)	2	
Lower Extremities**	Inspects and palpates left leg (1 point) Inspects and palpates right leg (1 point) Checks motor, sensory, and distal circulation (1 point/leg)	4	
Upper Extremities	Inspects and palpates left arm (1 point) Inspects and palpates right arm (1 point) Checks motor, sensory, and distal circulation (1 point/arm)	4	
Posterior Thorax/Lumbar** and Buttocks	Inspects and palpates posterior thorax (1 point) Inspects and palpates lumbar and buttocks area (1 point)	2	
Identifies and treats minor wounds/fractures appropriately (1 point each)		2	
	SECONDARY SURVEY SUB-TOTAL	23	

CRITICAL CRITERIA

____ Failure to initiate or call for transport of the patient within 10 minute time limit
____ Failure to take or verbalize infection control precautions
____ Failure to immediately establish and maintain spinal protection
____ Failure to provide high concentration of oxygen
____ Failure to evaluate and find all presented conditions of airway, breathing, and circulation (shock)
____ Failure to appropriately manage/provide airway, breathing, hemorrhage control or treatment for shock
____ Failure to differentiate patient's needing transportation versus continued on-scene survey
____ Does other detailed physical examination before assessing & treating threats to airway, breathing & circulation

You must factually document your rationale for checking any of the above critical items on the reverse side of this form.

National Registry of Emergency Medical Technicians
Paramedic Practical Examination

VENTILATORY MANAGEMENT (ET)

Candidate: _____ Examiner: _____

Date: _____ Signature: _____

NOTE: If candidate elects to initially ventilate with BVM attached to reservoir and oxygen, full credit must be awarded for steps denoted by "**" so long as first ventilation is delivered within initial 30 seconds.

	Possible Points	Points Awarded
Takes or verbalizes infection control precautions	1	
Opens the airway manually	1	
Elevates tongue, inserts simple adjunct [either oropharyngeal or nasopharyngeal airway]	1	
NOTE: Examiner now informs candidate no gag reflex is present and patient accepts adjunct		
**Ventilates patient immediately with bag-valve-mask device unattached to oxygen	1	
**Hyperventilates patient with room air	1	
NOTE: Examiner now informs candidate that ventilation is being performed without difficulty		
Attaches oxygen reservoir to bag-valve-mask device and connects to high-flow oxygen regulator [12–15 liters/min.]	1	
Ventilates patient at a rate of 10–20/min. and volumes of at least 800ml	1	
NOTE: After 30 seconds, examiner auscultates and reports breath sounds are present and equal bilaterally and medical control has ordered intubation. The examiner must now take over ventilation.		
Directs assistant to hyperventilate patient	1	
Identifies/selects proper equipment for intubation	1	
Checks equipment for: —Cuff leaks (1 point) —Laryngoscope operational and bulb tight (1 point)	2	
NOTE: Examiner to remove OPA and move out of the way when candidate is prepared to intubate		
Positions head properly	1	
Inserts blade while displacing tongue	1	
Elevates mandible with laryngoscope	1	
Introduces ET tube and advances to proper depth	1	
Inflates cuff to proper pressure and disconnects syringe	1	
Directs ventilation of patient	1	
Confirms proper placement by auscultation bilaterally and over epigastrium	1	
NOTE: Examiner to ask "If you had proper placement, what would you expect to hear?"		
Secures ET tube [may be verbalized]	1	

CRITICAL CRITERIA

TOTAL 19 [ ]

____ Failure to initiate ventilations within 30 seconds after applying gloves or interrupts ventilations for greater than 30 seconds at any time

____ Failure to take or verbalize infection control precautions

____ Failure to voice and ultimately provide high oxygen concentrations [at least 85%]

____ Failure to ventilate patient at rate of at least 10/minute

____ Failure to provide adequate volumes per breath [maximum 2 errors/minute permissable]

____ Failure to hyperventilate patient prior to intubation

____ Failure to successfully intubate within 3 attempts

____ Using teeth as a fulcrum

____ Failure to assure proper tube placement by auscultation bilaterally **_and_** over the epigastrium

____ If used, stylette extends beyond end of ET tube

____ Inserts any adjunct in a manner dangerous to patient

You must factually document your rationale for checking any of the above critical items on the reverse side of this form.

VENTILATORY MANAGEMENT (EOA)

Candidate: _____   Examiner: _____
Date: _____   Signature: _____

NOTE: If candidate elects to initially ventilate with BVM attached to reservoir and oxygen, full credit must be awarded for steps denoted by "**" so long as first ventilation is delivered within initial 30 seconds.

	Possible Points	Points Awarded
Takes or verbalizes infection control precautions	1	
Opens the airway manually	1	
Elevates tongue, inserts simple adjunct [either oropharangeal or nasopharangeal airway]	1	
NOTE: Examiner now informs candidate no gag reflex is present and patient accepts adjunct		
**Ventilates patient immediately with bag-valve-mask device unattached to oxygen	1	
**Hyperventilates patient with room air	1	
NOTE: Examiner now informs candidate that ventilation is being performed without difficulty		
Attaches oxygen reservoir to bag-valve-mask device and connects to high-flow oxygen regulator [12–15 liters/min.]	1	
Ventilates patient at a rate of 10–20/min. and volumes of at least 800ml	1	
NOTE: After 30 seconds, examiner auscultates and reports breath sounds are present and equal bilaterally and medical control has ordered placement of an EOA. The examiner must now take over ventilation.		
Directs assistant to hyperventilate patient	1	
Identifies/selects proper equipment	1	
Assembles airway	1	
Tests cuff	1	
Inflates mask	1	
Lubricates tube [may be verbalized]	1	
NOTE: Examiner to remove OPA and move out of way when candidate is prepared to insert EOA		
Positions head properly with neck in neutral or slightly flexed position	1	
Grasps tongue and mandible and elevates	1	
Inserts tube in same direction as curvature of pharynx	1	
Advances tube until mask sealed against face	1	
Ventilates patient while maintaining tight mask seal	1	
Directs confirmation of proper placement by auscultation bilaterally and over epigastrium	1	
Inflates cuff to proper pressure and disconnects syringe	1	
Continues ventilation of patient	1	
NOTE: Examiner to ask "If you had proper placement, what would you expect to hear?"		

TOTAL   21   [ ]

CRITICAL CRITERIA

____ Failure to initiate ventilations within 30 seconds after applying gloves or interrupts ventilations for greater than 30 seconds at any time
____ Failure to take or verbalize infection control precautions
____ Failure to voice and ultimately provide high oxygen concentrations [at least 85%]
____ Failure to ventilate patient at rate of at least 10/minute
____ Failure to provide adequate volumes per breath [maximum 2 errors/minute permissible]
____ Failure to hyperventilate patient prior to placement of the EOA
____ Failure to successfully place the EOA within 3 attempts
____ Failure to assure proper tube placement by auscultation bilaterally **_and_** over the epigastrium
____ Inserts any adjunct in a manner dangerous to patient

You must factually document your rationale for checking any of the above critical items on the reverse side of this form.

National Registry of Emergency Medical Technicians
Advanced Level Practical Examination

INTRAVENOUS THERAPY

Candidate: _____   Examiner: _____

Date: _____   Signature: _____

Time Start: _____ Time End: _____

	Possible Points	Points Awarded
Checks selected IV fluid for: —Proper fluid (1 point) —Clarity (1 point)	2	
Selects appropriate catheter	1	
Selects proper administration set	1	
Connects IV tubing to the IV bag	1	
Prepares administration set [fills drip chamber and flushes tubing]	1	
Cuts or tears tape [at any time before venipuncture]	1	
Takes/verbalizes infection control precautions [prior to venipuncture]	1	
Applies tourniquet	1	
Palpates suitable vein	1	
Cleanses site appropriately	1	
Performs venipuncture —Inserts stylette (1 point) —Notes or verbalizes flashback (1 point) —Occludes vein proximal to catheter (1 point) —Removes stylette (1 point) —Connects IV tubing to catheter (1 point)	5	
Releases tourniquet	1	
Runs IV for a brief period to assure patent line	1	
Secures catheter [tapes securely or verbalizes]	1	
Adjusts flow rate as appropriate	1	
Disposes/verbalizes disposal of needle in proper container	1	

CRITICAL CRITERIA   TOTAL 21 [ ]

_____ Exceeded the 6 minute time limit in establishing a patent and properly adjusted IV
_____ Failure to take or verbalize infection control precautions prior to performing venipuncture
_____ Contaminates equipment or site without appropriately correcting situation
_____ Any improper technique resulting in the potential for catheter shear or air embolism
_____ Failure to successfully establish IV within 3 attempts during 6 minute time limit
_____ Failure to dispose/verbalize disposal of needle in proper container

You must factually document your rationale for checking any of the above critical items on the reverse side of this form.

National Registry of Emergency Medical Technicians
Advanced Level Practical Examination

SPINAL IMMOBILIZATION
(SEATED PATIENT)

Candidate: _____ Examiner: _____

Date: _____ Signature: _____

Time Start: _____ Time End: _____

	Possible Points	Points Awarded
Takes or verbalizes infection control precautions	1	
Directs assistant to place/maintain head in neutral, in-line position	1	
Directs assistant to maintain manual immobilization of head	1	
Assesses motor, sensory, and distal circulation in extremities	1	
Applies appropriately sized extrication collar	1	
Positions the immobilization device behind the patient	1	
Secures device to the patient's torso	1	
Evaluates torso fixation and adjusts as necessary	1	
Evaluates and pads behind the patient's head as necessary	1	
Secures patient's head to the device	1	
Reassesses motor, sensory, and distal circulation in extremities	1	
Verbalizes moving the patient to a long board properly	1	
TOTAL	**12**	

CRITICAL CRITERIA

____ Did not immediately direct or take manual immobilization of the head

____ Releases or orders release of manual immobilization before it was maintained mechanically

____ Patient manipulated or moved excessively causing potential spinal compromise

____ Did not complete immobilization of the torso prior to immobilizing the head

____ Device moves excessively up, down, left, or right on patient's torso

____ Torso fixation inhibits chest rise resulting in respiratory compromise

____ Head immobilization allows for excessive movement

____ Upon completion of immobilization, head is not in neutral, in-line position

You must factually document your rationale for checking any of the above critical items on the reverse side of this form.

National Registry of Emergency Medical Technicians
Advanced Level Practical Examination

RANDOM BASIC SKILLS
BLEEDING—WOUNDS—SHOCK

Candidate: _____   Examiner: _____

Date: _____   Signature: _____

Time Start: _____ Time End: _____

	Possible Points	Points Awarded
Takes or verbalizes infection control precautions	1	
Applies direct pressure to the wound	1	
Elevates the extremity	1	
Applies pressure dressing to the wound	1	
Bandages wound		1
NOTE: The examiner must now inform the candidate that the wound is still continuing to bleed. The second dressing does not control the bleeding.		
Locates and applies pressure to the appropriate arterial pressure point	1	
NOTE: The examiner must indicate that the victim is in compensatory shock.		
Applies high concentration oxygen	1	
Properly positions patient (supine with legs elevated)	1	
Prevents heat loss (covers patient as appropriate)	1	
NOTE: The examiner must indicate that the victim is in profound shock. Medical control has ordered application and inflation of the Pneumatic Anti-shock Garment.		
Removes clothing or checks for sharp objects	1	
Quickly assesses areas that will be under the PASG	1	
Positions PASG with top of abdominal section at or below last set of ribs	1	
Secures PASG around patient	1	
Attaches hoses	1	
Begins inflation sequence (examiner to stop inflation at 15 mm Hg)	1	
Checks blood pressure	1	
Verbalizes when to stop inflation sequence	1	
Operates PASG to maintain air pressure in device	1	
Reassesses vital signs	1	

CRITICAL CRITERIA

TOTAL   19   [ ]

_____ Failure to take or verbalize infection control precautions

_____ Did not apply high concentration of oxygen

_____ Applies tourniquet before attempting other methods of hemorrhage control

_____ Did not control hemorrhage or attempt to control hemorrhage in a timely manner

_____ Inflates abdominal section of PASG before the legs

_____ Did not reassess patient's vital signs after PASG inflation

_____ Places PASG on inside-out

_____ Allows deflation of PASG after inflation

_____ Positions PASG above level of lowest rib

You must factually document rationale for checking any of the above critical items on the reverse side of this form.

National Registry of Emergency Medical Technicians
Advanced Level Practical Examination

RANDOM BASIC SKILLS
LONG BONE IMMOBILIZATION

Candidate: _____   Examiner: _____

Date: _____   Signature: _____

Time Start: _____ Time End: _____

	Possible Points	Points Awarded
Takes or verbalizes infection control precautions	1	
Directs application of manual stabilization	1	
Assesses motor, sensory, and distal circulation	1	
NOTE: Examiner acknowledges present and normal		
Measures splint	1	
Applies splint	`1	
Immobilizes joint above fracture	1	
Immobilizes joint below fracture	1	
Secures entire injured extremity	1	
Immobilizes hand/foot in position of function	1	
Reassesses motor, sensory, and distal circulation	1	
NOTE: Examiner acknowledges present and normal		
TOTAL	**10**	

CRITICAL CRITERIA

____ Grossly moves injured extremity

____ Did not immobilize adjacent joints, injury, or limb

____ Did not reassess motor, sensory, and distal circulation **after** splinting

You must factually document your rationale for checking any of the above critical items on the reverse side of this form.

National Registry of Emergency Medical Technicians
Advanced Level Practical Examination

RANDOM BASIC SKILLS
TRACTION SPLINTING

Candidate: _____   Examiner: _____

Date: _____   Signature: _____

Time Start: _____   Time End: _____

	Possible Points	Points Awarded
Takes or verbalizes infection control precautions	1	
Directs manual stabilization of injured leg	1	
Directs application of manual traction	1	
Assesses motor, sensory, and distal circulation	1	
NOTE: Examiner acknowledges present and normal		
Prepares/adjusts splint to proper length	1	
Positions splint at injured leg	1	
Applies proximal securing device (e.g. ischial strap)	1	
Applies distal securing device (e.g. ankle hitch)	1	
Applies mechanical traction	1	
Positions/secures support straps	1	
Re-evaluates proximal/distal securing devices	1	
Reassesses motor, sensory, and distal circulation	1	
NOTE: Examiner acknowledges present and normal		
NOTE: Examiner must ask candidate how he/she would prepare for transport		
Verbalizes securing torso to long board to immobilize hip	1	
Verbalizes securing splint to long board to prevent movement of splint	1	

CRITICAL CRITERIA
TOTAL   14

_____ Loss of traction at any point after it is assumed

_____ Did not reassess motor, sensory, and distal circulation **after** splinting

_____ The foot is excessively rotated or extended after splinting

_____ Did not secure ischial strap **before** taking traction

_____ Final immobilization failed to support femur or prevent rotation of injured leg

> **NOTE:**   If Sagar is used without elevating the leg, application of manual traction is not necessary. Candidate will be awarded 1 point as if manual traction were applied.
>
> **NOTE:**   If the leg is elevated at all, manual traction must be applied before elevating the leg. The ankle hitch may be applied before elevating the leg and used to pull manual traction.

You must factually document your rationale for checking any of the above critical items on the reverse side of this form.

RANDOM BASIC SKILLS
SPINE IMMOBILIZATION
(LYING PATIENT)

Candidate: _____   Examiner: _____

Date: _____   Signature: _____

Time Start: _____ Time End: _____

	Possible Points	Points Awarded
Takes or verbalizes infection control precautions	1	
Directs assistant to move patient's head to the neutral in-line position	1	
Directs assistant to maintain manual immobilization of head	1	
Evaluates motor, sensory, and distal circulation in extremities	1	
Applies cervical collar	1	
Positions immobilization device appropriately	1	
Moves patient onto device without compromising the integrity of the spine	1	
Applies padding to voids between the torso and the boards as necessary	1	
Immobilizes torso to the device	1	
Evaluates and pads under the patient's head as necessary	1	
Immobilizes the patient's head to the device	1	
Secures legs to the device	1	
Secures patient's arms to the board	1	
Reassesses motor, sensory, and distal circulation	1	

TOTAL   14

CRITICAL CRITERIA

____ Did not immediately direct manual immobilization of head

____ Orders release or manual immobilization before it was maintained mechanically

____ Did not complete immobilization of the torso prior to immobilizing the head

____ Device excessively moves up, down, left, or right on patient's torso

____ Head immobilization allows for excessive movement

____ Head is not immobilized in the neutral in-line position

____ Patient moved excessively causing potential spinal compromise

____ Did not reassess motor, sensory, and distal circulation **after** immobilization

You must factually document your rationale for checking any of the above critical items on the reverse side of this form.